Real
Food
Has
Curves

ALSO BY BRUCE WEINSTEIN AND MARK SCARBROUGH

The Ultimate Ice Cream Book

The Ultimate Party Drink Book

The Ultimate Candy Book

The Ultimate Shrimp Book

The Ultimate Brownie Book

The Ultimate Potato Book

Cooking for Two

The Ultimate Muffin Book

The Ultimate Chocolate Cookie Book

The Ultimate Frozen Dessert Book

The Ultimate Peanut Butter Book

The Ultimate Cook Book: 900 New Recipes,
Thousands of Ideas

Grill Thrills!

Pizza: Grill It, Bake It, Love It!

Cooking Know-How

Ham: An Obsession with the Hindquarter

Real Food Has Curves

How to Get Off Processed Food, Lose Weight, and Love What You Eat

With More Than 100 Recipes

~~~~~~~~~~~~~~~~~

Bruce Weinstein

AND

Mark Scarbrough

PHOTOGRAPHS BY Nisha Sondhe

Ⓖ

GALLERY BOOKS

New York London Toronto Sydney

G

Gallery Books
A Division of Simon & Schuster, Inc.
1230 Avenue of the Americas
New York, NY 10020

First Gallery Books hardcover edition May 2010.

Gallery Books and colophon are trademarks of Simon & Schuster, Inc.

For information about special discounts for bulk purchases, please contact Simon & Schuster Special Sales at 1-866-506-1949 or business@simonandschuster.com.

The Simon & Schuster Speakers Bureau can bring authors to your live event. For more information or to book an event, contact the Simon & Schuster Speakers Bureau at 1-866-248-3049 or visit our website at www.simonspeakers.com.

Manufactured in the United States of America

10 9 8 7 6 5 4 3 2 1

Library of Congress Cataloging-in-Publication Data

Weinstein, Bruce, 1960–
   Real food has curves : how to get off processed food, lose weight, and love what you eat with over 100 recipes / by Bruce Weinstein and Mark Scarbrough; photographs by Nisha Sondhe. — 1st Gallery Books hardcover ed.
       p.   cm.
   1. Reducing diets—Recipes.   2. Food—Psychological aspects.   I. Scarbrough, Mark. II. Title.
       RM222.2.W3285   2010
       641.5'63—dc22
2009047194

ISBN 978-1-4391-6038-1
ISBN 978-1-4391-6932-2 (ebook)

Contents

Welcome!

By dumping the overly processed stuff, relishing what you eat, and never fearing food again, you will feel better, lose weight, and most importantly, be satisfied.

Sounds great, right? Because in all honesty we're not satisfied—although we can eat whenever we want: rip open a bag of this or a box of that, cook a meal by assembling it from premade parts, eat it hot, eat it later, take it out, call it in, sit down and be served, put it in a doggy bag and have it right at hand anytime, day or night.

We can do all this and remain unsatisfied because the food's not real. It's processed, packaged, ridiculously sweet, unbelievably salty, mass-produced in such plummeting quality that it's had to be shellacked with fat and artificial junk just to make it palatable—not to mention pumped with preservatives and emulsifiers to keep it on the shelf well into the next Ice Age, all while fooling us into believing it's almost fresh.

Almost. That's the deal we've struck: a half-baked attempt to jog our memories about some real food we once had. But elves don't make cookies. Uncle Ben doesn't convert rice. And Mrs. Baird doesn't bake bread. Instead, marketing characters—or the corporations behind them—have given us strawberry pudding doped with artificial strawberry flavor, tomato juice loaded with more sodium than a cheeseburger, and microwavable chicken dinners laced with high-fructose corn syrup.

These fake-out flavors, fats, and additives give us little satisfaction. But boy, do we keep trying! As our friend Leslie Fink, the head nutritionist for weightwatchers.com, puts it, "When you're hungry and/or craving, if nothing satisfies you, you tend to keep eating until you get what you need—and that might be way past satiety."[1]

It's time to stop eating the fake stuff and start getting what we need.

The Road to Hell Is Paved With . . .

Fake food. Over the past few decades, as life moved more quickly, we gave up ripe vegetables for canned ones, tossed out sweet/tart orange juice for pasteurized concentrate, passed on the crunchy bread in favor of the gummy presliced stuff, traded steaks for boil-in-a-bag dinners, and gave up real desserts in favor of supersweet snacks that made us feel ridiculously overfed but definitely disappointed.

Despite our best intentions, we misled our stomachs, feeding them a bunch of artificial flavors, sweeteners, and additives that gave us a head rush without any deeper contentment. Our brains may not know an artificial sweetener from a real one, a mess of tasteless trans fats from a better fat, or a wad of processed apple pie filling from some freshly sliced apples and honey. That's because our brains process sensory information (*sweet! sour!*) and then can reward us for finding food that's not necessarily the best. We've let those up-top neurons override the ones in our bellies.

Did you know we've got a separate nervous system down there? It's made of neurons that operate with serotonin, dopamine, and the other chemicals also at work in our heads. Called the enteric nervous system, it has a profound effect on how we feel, how we eat, and maybe even how much we eat.

Having lost sight of real food and its true satisfaction, we've gained weight. Lots of it.[2] Upward of 65 percent of all Americans are either overweight or obese.[3] We're now in danger of what's inelegantly called the modern diseases: diabetes, clogged arteries, and even bad knees.

Let's be clear: eating fake food doesn't cause these problems; eating too much does. But fake food is so prevalent, cheap, and abundant that we've indeed gained weight, not because of it, but by means of it. In the end, it's not that we love food too much. It's that we love it too little.

Chances are, you've heard that one before—and tried to act on it. Ever walked into a supermarket and thought, *I'm going to eat better from now on*? Maybe you loaded your cart with whole-grain crackers, fish fillets, and asparagus. And then what? You got a few vaguely satisfying meals out of it before you thought, *Hey, life's too short for this.*

Resolutions aren't plans. They're flirtations with deprivation. You tried to say *no* to the huge world of less-than-the-best food until you couldn't say it anymore.

That's not real change. For that, you need a real plan.

You're holding it in your hands.

The Way Back

It's time to rediscover real food: curvy, voluptuous, juicy, sweet. And sexy, too. You don't really want boxes, mixes, or frozen entrées, all right angles and marketing scrawl, with a host of fake-outs lurking inside. You want ripe, gorgeous tomatoes; chicken with a crisp, brown skin; and a fruit crisp with a fulfilling allure far beyond the sweetener used to make it. So don't wait a moment longer. Step off on a journey to what truly satisfies.

Yes, you'll lose weight. But if you find yourself obsessing about a little cream in a skillet, you've mistaken this plan for some horrid diet. If you look in your fridge this week and wonder what you should toss out, you're getting too far ahead. Step back, take a deep breath, and continue with us.

How long will the plan take? Probably about ten weeks. But in reality, go at your own pace. Your health, happiness, and waistline may have suffered over the years, but you can't change the world overnight. Rome wasn't built in a day. Dinner, either.

If you want to slow down and really settle into one of the steps, good for you for knowing what you need. If you've sailed through and are ready to move on, good for you, too. Part of the reward is the journey itself. Well, that and a healthier body.

But to give you a better idea of where you're headed, here's a bird's-eye view of the seven steps:

Step 1: Learn the secrets to satisfaction.
Rediscover the basic pleasure of food by uncovering the real reasons you eat. Plan on spending about a week here, really settling into the ideas, which might seem simple at first but are in fact revolutionary.

Step 2: Make informed choices.
Learn how to recognize and savor real food. Some of these changes are a little more dramatic. Here's where you really come to terms with what's real and what's not. Spend about two weeks here, erasing old patterns to create new ones.

Step 3: Relish what you eat.
Understand why a diet is never the solution—and how our abundance is as much a curse as a blessing. Stick with these ideas for about a week.

Step 4: Detox your palate from useless salt, fat, and sugars.
Participate in a mini program to reorient your whole sense of taste. You're not going to get away from fat, salt, and sugars; you're going to demand they give you more flavor. Spend two weeks here and complete the program with a real, satisfying burger.

Step 5: Take the long view.
Dive into a week of attitude adjustments and real-world solutions that will encourage you to eat freely but mindfully.

Step 6: Upgrade your choices.
Spend a good two weeks learning how to find real food in the world around you.

Step 7: Treat yourself well.
Finally, the last week will round out your journey with a short course on the three ways you can treat yourself better every day: breakfast, snacks, and dessert.

All these steps include recipes—because nothing solidifies success like a good meal. Will you be cooking? Yes, more than you may have been. That's a key part of finding real food: preparing it. But a good meal is the best reward for hard work. Plus a happier, healthier you, of course.

We're All in This Together

Bruce and I needed this plan. Maybe it was the fault of our careers as busy food writers: sixteen cookbooks in ten years, not to mention our work as contributing editors to *Eating Well*, monthly columnists for weightwatchers.com, and frequent contributors to a host of food magazines, such as *Cooking Light* and *Fine Cooking*. Plus, we each come from cultures where food has always been a pretty big deal: Bruce (the chef) from a New York Jewish family and I (the writer) from a Texas Baptist one.

Truth be told, we didn't eat very well. So we gained weight. Not all at once, but over the years. There was just so much food around. I swear, one skillet in our kitchen hasn't been cool for a solid year.

Which means that we're just extreme versions of almost everyone else. Your pantry, your refrigerator—they're probably pretty well stocked. And if you need anything, there's a convenience store nearby, or a grocery store down the street, or a break room with vending machines, all bigger versions of your pantry and refrigerator.

Chances are, you're also near plenty of those enormous pantries of ready-to-eat meals we call restaurants. According to the National Restaurant Association, there are 945,000 of them in the United States.[4] We're surrounded by food. And eat too much. But not enough real food. And so eat even more.[5]

Bruce and I have spent the last year or so figuring out how to get back on an even keel. We made some small changes, then took bigger steps, all based on what we'd learned working for so many wellness publications.

Did we falter? Of course! But we whittled away at the problem until we were eating better and finding ourselves thinner, healthier, and more content. We couldn't ask for much more.

Because that's what it's all about: not real food per se, but better health and happiness. It's time to relish life, lose weight, and feel better. So *bon appétit*! *Tutti a tavola a mangiare*! And いらっしゃいませ![6]

Let's take the first step.

Real
Food
Has
Curves

～～～～～～～

THE SEVEN-STEP PLAN

STEP

1

Learn the Secrets to Satisfaction

WHAT WILL YOU DO?
Bite into a tasty peach
Connect memory to taste
Eat with several senses at once
Relish chewing

~~~~~~~~~~~~~~~~~

WHAT WILL YOU DISCOVER?
The complexity of our sense of taste
Flavor overtones
The necessity—and the trap—of a bolus
The basic textures of food

Eat a Peach

A ripe, irresistible peach is one of nature's better pleasures. Our first step is to celebrate it.

How do you find a great peach? Begin with your nose. If a peach doesn't smell like anything, it won't taste like anything. Search for that tantalizing fragrance. The best peach might not be the first one that comes to hand. Dig in the bin; smell the peaches one by one, particularly at the ends where their stems once were.

Got one with an unbelievable perfume? Look at it for a second. See that rosy blush over the dappled yellow? That's a sign you've chosen well.

Now gently squeeze the fruit. Although it's heavy to the hand, there's a delicate give beneath the skin—nothing squishy, just a little fragile, stocked with juice.

Once you've chosen (and paid for!) that peach, take a bite. Don't be shy. The juice bursts from the pulp, pooling in the corners of your mouth.

Chew a few times, then gently push what's in your mouth up against your hard palate, the roof of your mouth right behind your front teeth. Take a slow breath to draw in that sweet fragrance.

Swallow and take another bite. Because the miracle wasn't really that peach. It's what happened to you. You just took a step away from all that is processed, packaged, low nutrition, and poor quality. You just started down the road to enjoying food more, weighing less, and being more content with your life.

All that from tasting a peach? Absolutely.

Taste: A Seriously Underrated Sense

When we taste something wonderful, we experience some familiar physical reactions: the saliva in our mouths and a gurgle in our stomachs. But other, less familiar reactions are even more important: released chemicals in our brains set us up for both anticipation and its coming fulfillment in the neurons all along our digestive tracks, from our mouths to our stomachs and beyond.[1] If we take into account the run of chemical changes among those receptors, as well as the targeted preparations from our brains to our pancreases, taste's only rival may well be sexual arousal.

We don't even need a peach. If we imagine it, our brains instantly release those chemicals that drive us to find one and relish it. MRI scans prove that when we think of a specific food, our brains light up *the same way* they do when we're eating it.[2]

As you were reading about our perfect peach, you probably started salivating. Your brain was just doing its job: priming you for a peach although there were none in sight, not the slightest whiff of the fruit, just some words on a page.

Go Get Some Peaches

Put down this book and fulfill that desire. But don't just get one. Get a bunch. After you've tasted that peach to find the ways it connects to deeper pleasures in your mind, try one or both of these recipes.

Don't worry about changing any other food choices in your life. Keep doing what you're doing. Just focus on that peach—as well as these ways to upgrade its flavors. You'll notice that the recipes at the start of our journey are simple. We want to focus on tasting elemental flavors.

And one more thing: since you're going to be doing some cooking on your journey to real food, Bruce and I should offer you a few tips for kitchen success:

1. Before you begin a recipe, read it through, headnotes and all.

2. In general, Bruce's recipes call for ingredients the way you find them at your supermarket (for example, *2 celery stalks*). However, when less than a whole is called for, the ingredient is measured out (like *¼ cup diced red onion*).

3. Before you put a pot over the fire, gather your ingredients and put them out on the counter.

4. Make sure you've prepared the ingredients themselves. If the recipe says *1 medium yellow onion, chopped*, it's telling you that chopping will not be a part of the recipe itself. In other words, chop before you cook. By the way, *chopped, diced,* and *minced* are not clichés but real directions:

- *Roughly chopped* yields uneven pieces up to 1 inch wide;
- *chopped,* slightly smaller but also more uniform pieces, about ¾ inch on each side;
- *cubed,* small, ½-inch cubes;
- *finely chopped,* smaller still but less precise, about ¼-inch pieces;
- *diced,* ¼-inch cubes; and
- *minced,* the smallest of all, less than ⅛ inch, usually made by rocking a knife through an ingredient.

5. It's better to make substitutions and changes the second time you make a recipe.

FRESH PEACH SALSA

There are no tomatoes here, just sweet peaches. Tomatoes are firmer and almost meatier; by contrast, peaches offer a luxurious richness. That said, if you can't find a good peach, go for plums, apricots, or nectarines. Try this easy salsa on top of a baked potato with a dollop of sour cream or alongside some rotisseried chicken picked up at the market. Keep connecting the taste of those peaches to pleasure in your brain.

1½ pounds ripe medium peaches, pitted and diced (about 4 or 5 peaches)

Up to 1 medium fresh jalapeño chile, seeded and minced

½ cup red bell pepper, seeded and diced (see Note)

½ cup red onion, diced

3 tablespoons minced cilantro leaves, 2½ tablespoons stemmed thyme leaves, or 2 tablespoons minced mint leaves

2 tablespoons lime juice

½ teaspoon ground cumin

½ teaspoon salt

Stir everything together in a serving bowl. If you want to make the salsa ahead of time, omit the salt and store the mixture, covered, in the fridge for up to 2 days. Salt will leach liquid from the mixture, turning it watery during storage—so stir in the salt at the last minute.

Note: To seed and core a bell pepper, stand it up on your cutting board with the stem end facing up. Holding the stem, use a large knife to slice one side off the pepper, leaving the seeds attached to the core. Continue making more slices around the pepper, always leaving the seeds and core intact. Once all the wedges have been removed around the pepper, slice off any white membranes on their insides, discard the core, and prepare the pepper as directed in the recipe.

MAKES 8 SERVINGS

POACHED PEACHES

A minimal amount of cooking highlights the fruit's natural sugars by concentrating the flavors. Try these poached peaches for a midafternoon snack, a dessert at night, or even breakfast in the mornings. (Store them in the fridge for up to three days.) Serve them warm (either fresh off the stove or reheated in the microwave) with some of the poaching liquid and a little plain yogurt on the side.

4 ripe but firm peaches, halved through the stem ends, the pits removed and discarded

⅔ cup white wine or unsweetened apple juice

Water

2½ tablespoons honey

1 cup regular or low-fat plain yogurt

1. Place the peach halves cut side down in a skillet. Pour in the wine or apple juice, then add just enough water to come halfway up the peach halves.

2. Drizzle the honey over the peaches and into the poaching liquid. Set the skillet over medium heat and bring to a simmer.

3. Cover, reduce the heat to low, and simmer just until the peaches are tender when prodded with the back of a flatware spoon, 8 to 10 minutes. Use a large, slotted spoon to transfer them cut side up to a platter or serving bowls. The skins may be loose, may even come off. You can remove them if you'd like (although they're fully edible, of course).

4. Crank up the heat to high and bring the liquid in the skillet to a full simmer. Continue cooking until the liquid has reduced down to about ½ cup, stirring occasionally. Set off the stove to cool for 5 to 10 minutes, then spoon this liquid over the peach halves. Top each serving with ¼ cup yogurt.

MAKES 4 SERVINGS

~~~~~

Remembrance of Food Past

When I was a kid, my family vacationed in Colorado. One of my fondest memories was of our annual hunt for fresh, pan-fried trout. We'd look for the perfect little restaurant: family-owned, never hyped, lots of booths.

Even today, I remember the sizzle from the kitchen after our order was placed. And I distinctly remember the year I was old enough to get my own trout. I gingerly peeled back the skin to find the tender meat inside. I felt like such a grown-up!

Decades later, I'm driven to find and relish trout. Bruce roasts it some evenings with herbs layered in the belly. It's invariably satisfying, a link to my childhood.

That's the true power of taste. It isn't just in our mouths. It's mostly in our memories.

When we bite into something—already primed with chemical anticipation—our taste buds pick up various flavor molecules (like natural sugars or sour acids), then ping neurons in our brains keyed to those very molecules. One taste bud is saying to one neuron, *Here's something you like.* Except everyone's talking at once. Constantly. And insistently.

Plus, it's not just a set of person-to-person calls between taste buds and neurons; it's a convocation of conference calls. Our taste buds first ring up neurons at the base of our brains, near the structures that regulate basic life functions like sleeping and breathing. Those neurons then ring up others in higher level structures, the ones that stimulate pleasure and satisfaction—and most specifically, the ones keyed to our memories. So the pleasure we experience is based on a connection to the past.[3]

Taste strikes both at our cores (where we operate as living creatures) and also up at our cognitive centers (where we are thinking, feeling beings).[4] *Congratulations,* our brains tell us, *you found something that both supports life and makes it memorable.*

Memory stands at the center of our sense of taste—more than any other sense. Let's say your grandparents had a swing on an old oak tree. You probably don't sigh every time you pass an oak these days. But you probably do sigh every time you remember some wonderful dish your grandmother made. There it is: the essence of taste, that connection of memory and pleasure. It drives you to make food choices in the world around you.

But do you find real food, like that fresh trout sizzling in the skillet? No. Mostly, you find fish sticks, made from extruded, low-quality fish, fried in tasteless, heart-damaging oils—foods that don't satisfy because they connect inexactly and poorly to memories.

Which then drives you to try to find something that does. Unsatisfied but still stimulated, you search for more. And more. And more.[5] When all you want is a flavorful meal. Like this one:

HERB-STUFFED TROUT

Try this simple recipe for boneless, whole trout, a perfect, straightforward, and pleasurable dinner with nothing more than a green salad on the side.

Two 14- to 16-ounce boneless, cleaned trout

½ teaspoon salt

½ teaspoon freshly ground black pepper

Various herb sprigs, such as thyme, rosemary, parsley, oregano, tarragon, and/or dill (see Note)

1 medium lemon, very thinly sliced

1 tablespoon olive oil

1. Preheat the oven to 425°F.

2. Blot the trout dry with paper towels inside and out. Season the fish with both salt and pepper on the inside.

3. Divide the herbs and lemon slices between the two body cavities, sandwiching them closed to hold in the herbs and lemon slices.

4. Heat a large, oven-safe skillet over medium heat. A seasoned cast-iron skillet is really best. Swirl in the oil, then slip in the stuffed trout. Cook until the skin on one side has begun to get crisp, about 5 minutes.

5. Use a large spatula to turn the fish, then put the skillet in the oven and continue cooking until the meat will flake when gently pulled with a fork, about 8 more minutes.

Note: Good herb combinations include oregano and rosemary, thyme and parsley, tarragon and thyme, or parsley and dill. Plan on five to seven sprigs per trout (but in any case, no more than one rosemary spear per trout).

MAKES 4 SERVINGS
(CAN BE HALVED OR DOUBLED)

The Problem: Eating Without Tasting

Very early one morning last summer, Bruce and I were in the Hartford Airport, waiting to catch a flight to London. Checked in and through security, we found a place serving breakfast, ordered egg sandwiches, and took them to the gate. I soon caught myself eating like this: chew once or twice, still holding the sandwich near my mouth; chew a couple more times; the minute there's room, take another bite; chew some more; swallow a partial bite; keep holding the sandwich near my mouth; take another bite when there's room; swallow partially; and on and on.

It was hardly a pleasurable meal. Sometimes, food is just fuel. But in all honesty, Bruce and I eat like this more often than we'd like to admit. And we're not alone. Over the past year, we've watched people at the mall food court, in adult casual restaurants, and even in high-end restaurants eat exactly the same way: the fork poised over the food before a bite is gone, the next in before the last is out, a sort of unconscious conveyor belt of eating, a few chews and then more in the mouth, never a full swallow—and never much thought to what's happening on the plate.

The pleasure of food has been short-circuited; its connection to memory, almost nonexistent. Deep inside, we're waiting for it, primed and standing by, the brain rush in full gear. But since we're not finding satisfaction, we just keep eating.[6]

But here's the strange thing about that brain rush: it starts out at almost full blower. Remember those MRI scans that showed the mind lighting up at the mere thought of a peach? Everything's firing full out. However, our sense of pleasure doesn't get any more intense the more we eat. In fact, it lessens.

Thus, by the third bite of those breakfast sandwiches, Bruce and I weren't tasting anymore. We certainly weren't getting any measurable pleasure. We were just eating to scratch an itch in our heads. And eating. And eating. Until we'd forgotten the point. Which is to thrive and be content.

One Solution: Eating with All Our Senses

Let's go back to our peach. It was crucial to begin by experiencing a bit of real food with all our senses. We smelled that aroma, held the fruit in our hands, saw how beautiful it was, and heard its delicate crunch.

In other words, we tasted it fully. We took that crazy chemical dance in our heads and turned it into a slower, more elegant waltz by complicating those brain signals with more sensory input, forcing our minds to process even more information. That way, we got even more pleasure out of what we ate. We moved away from the chemical wash that is purely taste and pushed the experience into multiple senses, the better to enjoy it longer.

So here's to eating with all our senses. Can we every time? No. But can we most of the time? Yes. If we but take the time.

And there's the rub: time. Because eating just to fake ourselves out is efficient and quick. Relishing food takes time. It's passionate. It requires that we taste fully and deeply.

Every day, we come across a host of things we love but eat without thought: chocolate cookies, butter pecan ice cream, banana pudding. If tasting requires time, we have to learn to make these things a meal—or at least savor them.[7]

So here's a plan: no more eating on the run, in the car, on the train, while walking down the street, or while talking on the phone. If we're going to have an ice-cream cone, let's sit down and have one. If we're going to grab a chocolate cookie at the mall, let's order a cup of coffee, too, and stop to enjoy them both slowly, eating with all five senses.

Another Solution: Finding Flavor Overtones

The more memory connections we find in taste, the more pleasure we'll experience in food.

And as we begin to use all our senses to slow down how we taste, we'll begin to experience *flavor overtones*—faint flavors that ride up over the top of what we taste.

A processed egg sandwich at an airport will have few if any—and thus less pleasure bite per bite. Processed and packaged food lacks a range of overtones—because the fats are tasteless, the sugars are nothing but a vague notion of sweet, the salt is packed in with a heavy pour, and the flavors are ridiculously simplified.

By contrast, a nicely prepared breakfast of scrambled eggs, crunchy toast, and some fruit salad will have many overtones, each connected to its own, distinct flavor memory, a gorgeous dance that brings deeper satisfaction.

My mother loves vanilla, doubling the amount in any recipe. Her snickerdoodle cookies are redolent with the stuff! These days, I can catch a vanilla overtone in a glass of red wine or a slice of cantaloupe. It brings me more pleasure because it connects to more memories, most of the time not even consciously.

As you begin to taste more carefully and consciously, you'll begin to see how flavor overtones play an important part in satiety. (And you may begin to see that what you've been eating doesn't have many overtones at all.) Be on the lookout for these flavors:

Honey
Vanilla
Pineapple
Various herbs
Chiles
Licorice
Citrus
Lemon
Nuts of all sorts
Cinnamon
Yeast
Berries
Tea
Chocolate
Toast

As you slow down to relish food with all your senses, you'll find even more flavor overtones.[8] And that joy of discovery—not just the overtones but the sheer pleasure of discovery itself—will become increasingly essential to finding and relishing real food.

Fresh Is Best—*When Possible*

Questions of pleasure in food, of finding the best and enjoying it, sometimes call up a weird nostalgia for a blissful past when people supposedly ate right. Once upon a time, everyone walked out their doors, scooped up raw vegetables, took a bite out of a nearby cow, and went about their business.[9]

Um, no. New Englanders in January of any year before 1900 ate almost no fresh food. They couldn't. Not even eggs. Hens stop laying with the loss of daylight. Everything had to be preserved and cured—for survival's sake.

The same goes for that perfectly ripe peach. There are times when we have to buy a bag of frozen, unsweetened, sliced peaches. Are they the absolute best? No. But do they work? Definitely. They will taste luscious and light, particularly in recipes like this quick soup.

As you prepare one or both of these following recipes, think of a previous time when you had a great peach. Maybe it was just the other day when we were sampling that peach in and for itself! In any case, try to feel how one flavor is connected to a memory, even when encased among other, more complicated tastes. Relish those overtones, which then connect to still more memories and bring even more satisfaction.

CHILLED PEACH SOUP

Peaches aren't just a side dish or a dessert. Their natural sweetness can turn even simple dishes into intense pleasures. Serve this summery soup for lunch with a salad on the side—or make it the first course before some shrimp or chicken off the grill. By the way, when a recipe asks you to *whisk something*, it means you should use a whisk. *Stir* means to use a wooden spoon.

2 pounds ripe peaches, pitted and quartered (no need to peel)	One 4-inch cinnamon stick
4 cups water	½ cup white wine or nonalcoholic sparkling cider (see Note)
½ teaspoon ground cloves	½ cup low-fat yogurt or sour cream
½ teaspoon salt	¼ cup honey

1. Bring the peaches, water, cloves, salt, and cinnamon stick to a simmer in a large saucepan over medium-high heat.

2. Cover, reduce the heat to low, and simmer until the peaches are meltingly tender, about 12 minutes.

3. Fish out and discard the (hot!) cinnamon stick. Use a slotted spoon to transfer the peaches themselves to the canister of a blender or a food processor.

4. Return the saucepan to high heat and bring the liquid to a full simmer. Cook until that liquid has reduced to half its volume, about 8 minutes. Set aside to cool for 10 minutes.

5. Pour this liquid into the blender or the food processor. If you're working with a blender, cover it but remove the center knob on the lid and place a clean kitchen towel over the opening to prevent its spewing hot peach soup everywhere. If you're working with a food processor, remove the center of the large insertion tube on top and cover for the same reason. Blend or process until smooth.

6. Pour the puree into a large bowl. Whisk in the wine or nonalcoholic sparkling cider, yogurt or sour cream, and the honey. Chill for 1 hour, then cover and continue chilling for at least 4 hours or overnight.

Note: Although the soup tastes best if it chills overnight, it might also thicken up a bit. Stir it down to loosen it up. If that doesn't work, add a little more wine or sparkling cider, just a splash, to get it smooth again.

MAKES 6 SERVINGS

PEACH AND GOAT CHEESE QUESADILLAS

A little bit of fat (in this case, the creamy goat cheese) intensifies the peachy flavor dramatically. Don't worry about the calories— we're not using that much cheese. Besides, we want to focus on the pleasure of enticing food.

2 ounces soft goat cheese or chèvre, at room temperature

Four 8-inch fat-free whole wheat tortillas (see Note)

2 ripe peaches, pitted and thinly sliced

2 jarred roasted red bell peppers or pimientos, packed in water and drained, then cut into thin strips

Several dashes hot red pepper sauce, such as Tabasco sauce

1. Preheat the broiler, setting the oven rack about 4 to 6 inches from the heat source.

2. Divide and smear the goat cheese on one side of each of the tortillas, spreading it to within ¼ inch of the perimeter of each.

3. Top two of the smeared tortillas with the peach slices and red pepper strips. Dot with a few dashes of hot red pepper sauce, as much as you'd like for your heat preference.

4. Top each of these two tortillas with one of the other tortillas, cheese side down. Set the tortilla sandwiches on a large baking sheet and place under the broiler.

5. Cook until lightly browned, then turn with a large spatula. If a peach slice slips out, just stick it back in. Continue broiling until lightly browned on the other side. Transfer to a wire rack and cool for 5 minutes before slicing into pie-shaped wedges.

Note: Many fat-free tortillas are definitely real food: just flour and water without anything else in the mix.

MAKES 2 SERVINGS
(CAN BE DOUBLED OR TRIPLED FOR A FAMILY LUNCH)

Enjoy Every Bite

We should have known! While we were cutting our Peach and Goat Cheese Quesadillas into pie-shaped wedges, the processed and packaged food world was figuring out how to create a perfect bolus *(boh-luhs,* from the Latin *bolos,* meaning "clod").

Sounds like a disease, no? A bolus is the wad of food in our mouths when we chew, right before we swallow.

A bite of pound cake becomes a bolus quickly; a piece of celery, not so much—or not without a lot of chewing. In fact, celery may never become a true bolus, remaining a loose aggregate in the mouth. That's why we want to dunk it in a creamy dip. It softens the impact.

There's a range of effort required to get a bolus from foods. Pasta from refined, white flour becomes a bolus more easily than noodles from whole wheat flour. Ground meat? More quickly than steak. Cheese? More quickly than a pear—and much more quickly than an apple.

That said, all these things are real food. And they have a range of textures. Which is mostly how we experience boluses. When we talk about the texture of food, by and large we're talking about how quickly it becomes a bolus.

These days, we've lost the range. Most of what we eat is soft. It becomes a bolus very quickly. Think about fast food, packaged cookies, smoothies, or sugary breakfast cereals after they've sat in the milk for half a minute.

Whatever happened to chewing?

It Was Wiped Out by Design

When Bruce developed corporate recipes at a food marketing agency in New York City in the early nineties, he had many discussions with clients and management about getting food soft enough to become a bolus quickly and effortlessly. As he tells it, there were several reasons:

1. to get us sated before we realized the flavors in our food were absurdly elementary,

2. to get us full with minimal effort, and

3. to get us in and out of a restaurant's door as quickly as possible.

So how did he work to get a fast bolus? Three ways:

1. pump up the sugar,

2. load up the fat, or

3. do both.

Think of the sweet sauces in a chicken wrap from a fast-food restaurant. Think of fried foods: a sugar-laced batter that's stocked with fat from the deep-fryer.

All of which stops our well-warranted attempts to taste every bite.

The Chewless Society

Our jaws aren't what they used to be. Our ancestors ate a host of raw, tough, fibrous foods. As we began to cook over fire, we needed to chew our food fewer times per bite. Our jaws soon lost their girth.[10]

Chewing fewer times is pretty foundational to who we are as modern humans. It may well indicate our increased civilization: we're better than the animals because we cook; we don't tear and rend.

Too bad our brains still respond to chewing. We need it to be satisfied. The research is solid: people who chew more eat less.[11] Chewing more means more time at the table. And people who spend *more* time at the table tend to consume *fewer* calories than those who don't. What's more, children in families who spend *more* time at the table, who don't eat on the run, eat more fruits and vegetables (things that become boluses *less* quickly) as well as fewer snacks.[12]

As we chew, our taste buds send their signals up to our brains, which then send messages down the vagus nerve to the neurons that stretch along the enteric nervous system in our digestive tracks. By not chewing, we short-circuit that process. We swallow before we know it. We not only lose out on the pleasure of our food; but having misses cued to satiety, we're prone to be hungry in an hour or so.

Our grandmothers were right: chewing is the first step to good digestive health. It not only cuts down on gastric stress (those large boluses that land with a thud in our stomachs), but it also releases enzymes in our saliva that begin breaking down fiber, natural sugars, and fats—and in turn cause the release of various pleasure chemicals in our cranial *and* enteric nervous systems.

A wider range of textures will help us chew more, eat less, and be satisfied longer. We have to relish all the textures we can experience, including these:

Crunchy
Smooth
Chewy
Fibrous
Pulpy
Sticky
Slippery
Creamy
Grainy
Dense
Firm
Velvety
Hard
Marshmallowy
Snappy

A Chew Test—and Three Recipes

Experience for yourself the effect of excess sugar and fat on food and its ability to become a bolus.

First, you'll need to go to the store to buy a few things:

1. a can of pear halves packed in light syrup

2. a can of pear halves packed in juice or water

3. a fresh pear

4. a small piece of cheese, preferably a creamy cheese like Havarti or even blue cheese

While you're at the supermarket, glance down and pick up the ingredients for one or more of the following recipes, to further explore the range of textures in food.

Okay, on to the experiment. Set your selections out on the table and have a seat. First, sample the pear packed in juice or water, then the one packed in syrup. Feel the difference in your mouth. What texture does the extra sugar bring to the pear? A slight slipperiness?

Now take a bite from the fresh pear. Notice that crunch. Notice the more pressing way you have to work the food in your mouth. But is it buzzing? Are you salivating? Probably—and maybe more so than you were with the other two versions of the pear.

As to their tastes, if you had to rate the three in terms of fragrance, how would they stack up against one another? And in terms of texture? How are the three different? Does the sugar in the syrup mask flavors in any way?

Which one most quickly becomes a bolus? Which one is the easiest to swallow? Taste a little piece of cheese with a bite of the fresh pear. Besides the obvious shift in taste, how does the cheese, a high-fat food, change the chew of the fresh pear?

Sugar and fat dramatically alter chewing. They can modify it to good effect, adding more pleasure to what we eat (a crunchy cookie, a chicken breast browned in butter); but they can also go too far, mitigating chewing entirely, turning food into a soft, slippery bolus without any flavor overtones. They are dumped into processed and packaged foods precisely so you can swallow quickly, well before you realize the flavors are elementary, monochromatic, and uninteresting. There's only one cure for that: real food.

THYME AND GARLIC-ROASTED SHRIMP

All shrimp are sold by weight. Labels like jumbo or large are mere window dressing; shrimp are sized by how many make up a pound. They're also quite sweet—almost unbelievably so. But you won't know it unless you chew them well, letting the flavors develop bite by bite. What a reward is in store for you!

2 tablespoons olive oil

8 to 10 thyme sprigs

2 garlic cloves, quartered

2 pounds medium shrimp (30 per pound), peeled and deveined (see Note)

2 tablespoons white wine vinegar

½ teaspoon salt

½ teaspoon freshly ground black pepper

1. Pour the olive oil into a 9 x 13-inch baking dish or similarly sized roasting pan.

2. Add the thyme and garlic to the baking dish. Set the dish in the oven, then preheat the oven to 450°F for 15 minutes.

3. Add the shrimp, stir it all up a bit, then roast until pink and firm, about 8 minutes, tossing gently two or three times with a wooden spoon.

4. Remove the baking dish from the oven and stir in the vinegar, salt, and pepper.

Note: To peel a shrimp, turn it over so its legs face you, take the shrimp in both hands, and use your thumbs to pull the legs gently away from each other, tearing the shell down the middle of its underside. Peel back the shell, then grasp the very end of the tail, just at the feathery flippers, to pull the meat free. To devein it, place it on your work surface so the convex (arched) side faces up. Run a paring knife along the curve, slitting the meat only until the dark vein is revealed; use the tip of the knife to pick out the vein or rinse the shrimp to wash out the vein. Of course, you can always ask the person at your supermarket to do the job for you. Or buy already peeled and deveined shrimp right from the counter.

MAKES 4 SERVINGS

RATATOUILLE CASSEROLE

Roasting is the best way to keep the crunch and chew in vegetables. So Bruce has morphed a classic, soft stew of tomatoes and eggplant into a dinner with more tooth. For a fuller meal, melt some cheese on some crunchy bread under the broiler to go alongside it. Or set about 1 ounce of soft goat cheese in a bowl, then spoon a serving of the hot vegetable casserole on and around it.

2 medium tomatoes (about 1 pound), chopped

2 medium zucchini (about 1 pound), halved lengthwise and cut into ½-inch slices

2 small eggplants (about 1 pound), stemmed, quartered, and cut into ½-inch slices

1 large red onion, chopped

3 garlic cloves, minced

3 tablespoons olive oil

1 teaspoon minced oregano leaves or ½ teaspoon dried oregano

1 teaspoon stemmed thyme leaves or ½ teaspoon dried thyme

½ teaspoon salt

½ teaspoon freshly ground black pepper

1. Position a rack in the center of the oven and preheat to 375°F.

2. Toss all the ingredients in a large bowl, then pour them into a large, shallow roasting pan or oven-safe casserole.

3. Cover and bake for 45 minutes, stirring a few times.

4. Uncover and continue baking until the vegetables are tender, stirring frequently, about 15 minutes. Serve warm.

MAKES 6 SERVINGS

SALMON ROASTED WITH SALSA

This simple supper is guaranteed to get your mouth buzzing. The fish is silky and smooth, a delicious treat; but the fresh salsa stays a little crunchy, providing a contrast to the salmon.

Olive oil

One 1½-pound salmon fillet, skin on or off as you choose, left whole or cut the short way into 4 equal pieces

2 large tomatoes, cut into eight pieces each (about 1 pound total weight)

1 medium shallot, peeled and quartered

Up to 1 medium jalapeño chile, seeded and quartered

1 medium garlic clove, halved

2 tablespoons stemmed cilantro leaves (rinse them to remove any grit)

1 tablespoon lime juice

1½ teaspoons chile powder

½ teaspoon ground cumin

½ teaspoon salt

½ teaspoon freshly ground black pepper (see Note)

1. Dab a little oil on a crumpled paper towel and use it to grease a large baking sheet or oven roasting pan. Place the salmon fillet or fillets skin side down (or former skinned side down) in the pan. Set aside.

2. Place the tomatoes, shallot, chile, garlic, cilantro, lime juice, chile powder, cumin, salt, and pepper in a food processor fitted with the chopping blade. Pulse a few times until coarsely chopped. If you prefer a chunkier salsa or don't have a food processor, chop all these vegetables by hand, rocking a large knife through them repeatedly while they're on a cutting board.

3. Spoon the tomato salsa on top of the salmon, spreading the salsa to the sides. Spoon any extra around the fish. Now position a rack in the center of the oven and preheat to 400°F. Leave the topped salmon in the baking dish on the counter for 10 to 15 minutes while the oven preheats, so the flavors of the salsa permeate the fish.

4. Bake until hot, until the meat can be pulled into opaque, moist layers with a fork, about 20 minutes for individual pieces or 25 minutes if the fillet has been left whole. Let stand at room temperature for 5 minutes before serving.

Note: Over and over, these recipes call for *freshly ground black pepper*—simply because it tastes best. Buying whole black peppercorns and a pepper grinder is one small change that adds up to lots of flavor in your cooking. But how do you know how much is ½ teaspoon from that grinder? Do this experiment: make a small hash mark on the top of your grinder; starting from this point, grind pepper onto a cutting board until you get ¼ teaspoon. (Yes, this one time you'll have to scoop and measure.) Now that you know how many turns or cranks it takes to make ¼ teaspoon, do the math for all the other permutations: two times that many cranks for ½ teaspoon, four times that many cranks for 1 teaspoon, eight times that many cranks for 2 teaspoons.

MAKES 4 SERVINGS

~~~~~~

Putting Taste and Texture Together— or, the Sad Case of Burgers

A while back, Bruce and I had to get one of our computers fixed. From our house in the Litchfield hills of Connecticut, it's a good hour to a computer store. No problem—it was a warm, spring morning. We decided to take the day off.

Once we got the computer checked in, we had a few hours to ourselves. We thought we'd find a place for lunch.

Across the street, we spotted one of those so-called *adult casual* restaurants, the kind that specializes in burgers. We drove over and got on the list.

The place was packed: a twenty-minute wait on a run-of-the-mill weekday. Finally, our table was called and we were given menus like circus placards. But we bucked the forced fun and ordered simply: two cheeseburgers, no fries, two iced teas.

The moment the burgers were swept to our table, they were hard to resist: the tops of the buns slightly askew, lots of shredded lettuce, the red tomato peeking out. I set mine aright and took a bite.

It was very soft. I didn't need a drop to drink. The bun instantly balled up into a soft mass like whipped bread. Two chews and there wasn't much left.

The lettuce and tomato were tasteless, no flavor overtones at all. Yes, there was some crunch, but minimal, certainly nothing that required more than a chew or two. It was more like the notion of crunch.

I took another bite. I couldn't get over how soft it was—not velvety, but a little spongy. And sweet. Very sweet. But without any distinction as to what kind of sweet. Not like that peach with its various perfumes, a range of flavor notes. Instead, this registered as generic sweet. And unbelievably salty, too.

"I think I see a meat patty in there," Bruce said.

I picked at it with my fork. It pulled apart unattractively, stringy and slick. Despite being a ¼ inch thick, it was smooth, without much texture.

Yet I took another bite. And another. Bruce, too. Because that burger had pushed our appetites into overdrive. We downed our meal in less time than we had waited for the table. We paid and made it back to the mall—only to find ourselves eyeing the muffins in the food court an hour later. That's not being satisfied. That's being overfed, undersatisfied, and overweight. Not because of what we ate. But because of what went into what we ate.

How Real Food Becomes Fake

A burger could be consummately real food: lean ground beef, lots of chopped or sliced vegetables, and grains (in the bun, of course). Add a salad with crunchy veggies and there's a meal almost any nutritionist would like.

Except a burger barely exists as real food anymore. The beef is probably of poor quality, fairly tasteless but still greasy, a slick film on the lips.[13] It's probably been ground and preshaped in a facility hundreds of miles from the restaurant, then trucked in. And the patty may well include industrial filler, made by deodorizing and tenderizing ground snouts, cartilage, and even less savory bits with ammonia and other chemical shenanigans.

The lettuce? In our hydrator at home, it goes squishy in a week. But on those burgers, it's been prechopped, probably traveled interstate in a plastic bag, sealed for who knows how long, and stored in the fridge until someone was ready to open it and plop it on the patty—right under that sliced tomato which was most likely picked green and ripened with ethylene gas, an induced bit of red in an otherwise fibrous slice.

Cheese is an art, a lifetime of craft in every bite. And definitely real food. But the squares on our burgers? Merely shaped oil with a slight tang. Take a look at the single slices in the supermarket sometime. Why are they called *cheese food* and not *cheese*?

And finally, those alleged grains in the bun. They're barely there, refined until almost unrecognizable, then probably mixed with corn syrup as well as stabilizers, all to keep the buns fresh for weeks on end. What's more, that sugar pumped into the bun helps it melt on our tongues, the way sugar has a wont of doing. No need to chew. Just bite and dissolve, a bun version of a throat lozenge.

Can you believe they get us to wait in line for this stuff? It's all a consummate fake: unsatisfying yet quite elaborate (in many ways more so than a real burger), more like a reminder than the real thing. It goes down really quickly, fills us up, and leaves us hungry two hours later. We know what a real burger is. But we don't get it.

Still, there it is, the great modern marketing plan. So as long as we've enjoyed a real burger once in our lives, we'll keep searching for it, even through a host of poor imitators and stand-ins, none of which leads to any long-lasting satisfaction.

And it's not just burgers. It's the same with pizza. And chicken. And cookies. And chocolate. And cheese. And bread. On and on it goes—until we've long ago buried the real down under the fake and convinced ourselves that the poor-quality representation is the thing itself.

This is how we suffer. We're a country in an obesity epidemic, a country of chronic overeaters: in a constant flurry to find the real, eating too much, finding little to satisfy, and doing it all again.

One Way to Buck the Trend

All is not lost. There are ways to eat out without resorting to soft, tasteless food.

In general, look for a small restaurant where someone is not just cooking but actually creating dishes in the kitchen. Maybe it's a little bakery that serves sandwiches and salads in a strip mall by your home; maybe it's a nicer restaurant you've always wanted to try. It certainly doesn't have to be four-star dining, but you want a place without corporate recipe development. Need some recommendations? Check out websites like chowhound.com.

Sit back and make the meal an event. Don't rush off to the kids' soccer practice. Instead, get a glass of wine for a starter and have an espresso for dessert. Work on chewing the food. Savor it. Try to figure out its taste and texture, the various overtones. What herbs are in there? How does the taste change bite per bite?

And if chewing is necessary for satiety, here are some tips to getting extra texture in your meal:

✦ Ask for extra lettuce on the sandwich—or see if they have any crunchy lettuce back there, better than the squishy mesclun salad mix.

✦ Ask for a double portion of veggies.

✦ See if there are veggies included with another entrée you might like with yours. Look for roasted or sautéed choices, rather than those baked into casseroles or tricked out with too much cheese.

✦ Pick the whole-grain choices.

✦ Speak up. *What can I order that has lots of texture?* If the only answer is a list of things from the deep fryer, consider going elsewhere.

Find the flavor overtones, connect them to memory, discover more through chewing—then forget about it. Have a good conversation or enjoy your book. Be content with life and what sustains it: real food.

A Second Way to Buck the Trend

The other day, Bruce and I were working all morning on different projects: he was testing recipes for an *EatingWell* article; I was working on the scripts for a series of videos on the weightwatchers .com site. Sometime around 12:45, he called in to the study to see if I was ready to eat. To be honest, I hadn't even known it was lunchtime!

I came in to the kitchen and saw him dishing up a simple meal he'd made in less than twenty minutes: some whole wheat pasta with a sauce made from mild turkey sausage, shredded carrots, a diced hot chile, and some marjoram.

We sat down at the dining-room table and ate a bowl. We each even had a glass of beer. We found ourselves slowing down: savoring the meal and talking about our work, the incessant deadlines of two food writers making a go of it in a bad economy.

All the while, I loved the textures of the food he'd made: crunchy celery, soft onions, a little chew to the whole wheat pasta. That full range demanded chewing—which brought out the distinct elements of the dish: the spice of the chile, the full nose of the marjoram, the sweet carrots. And yes, the salty sausage, too—which spiked my hunger and made the dish more satisfying.

In the end, that lunch took longer to eat that it did to make. Forty minutes later, we both went back to work—and neither of us was eyeing any muffins by midafternoon.

Those burgers by the mall felt spartan. After all, we ordered no fries, no bacon, no bells or whistles.[14] Whereas our lunch at home was deeply satisfying, a wide range of tastes and textures, all prepared without much effort.

That's our goal: real food. The flavors spring forward yet also need time to develop. They demand to be tasted *and* chewed. They are simple, recognizable, and elemental. They satisfy.

SPAGHETTI WITH SAUSAGE, CARROTS, AND FRISÉE

Here's Bruce's lunch in a double size for a family meal. The tastes are still pretty straightforward, but there's a good range of textures. Savor them in every bite.

10 ounces dried whole wheat spaghetti

1 tablespoon olive oil

1 small yellow onion, chopped

6 ounces mild Italian sausage, any exterior casings removed

4 celery stalks, thinly sliced

4 medium carrots, peeled, then shredded through the large holes of a box grater

2 medium garlic cloves, minced

2 teaspoons minced marjoram or 1 teaspoon dried marjoram

1 teaspoon fennel seeds

½ teaspoon red pepper flakes

¼ teaspoon grated nutmeg

¼ teaspoon salt

1 cup dry white wine or dry vermouth (see Notes)

4 cups packed, chopped, cored frisée (about 2 small heads, see Notes)

¼ cup finely grated Parmigiano-Reggiano (see Notes)

1. Bring a large pot of water to a boil over high heat. Add the pasta, then stir a bit while it softens until it's all down in the simmering water. Continue cooking, stirring once in a while, until cooked through but with still a little bite in each piece. Drain in a colander set in the sink.

2. Heat a large skillet over medium heat, then swirl in the oil.

3. Add the onion; cook, stirring often just until the onion starts to soften, about 2 minutes.

4. Crumble in the sausage. Continue cooking until it loses its raw, pink color, stirring occasionally and breaking up any chunks, about 3 minutes.

5. Add the celery, carrot, and garlic; cook, stirring often, for 2 minutes. Why add them now, not before the sausage? So that they'll stay crunchy in the final dish.

6. Mix in the marjoram, fennel seeds, red pepper flakes, nutmeg, and salt for 20 seconds, just until aromatic. Then pour in the wine, and bring to a full simmer, scraping any browned stuff off the bottom of the skillet.

7. Once the wine has come to a full simmer, add the frisée and stir well for a minute or so while it wilts.

8. Stir in the drained spaghetti and the cheese. Toss a few times over the heat so that the spaghetti absorbs some of that sauce and warms up. Remove the skillet from the heat and stir a few times to make sure everything's mixed together.

Notes: Dry vermouth is a great alternative to white wine because once opened, it can stay on the shelf in a cool, dry place for several months.

Frisée is a slightly bitter green with long spidery tendrils. Look for tight heads with more white and pale yellow than green. If you can't find frisée, substitute curly endive or finely chopped escarole. To chop frisée, set it on your cutting board with the root end to the left or right. Beginning at the farthest point from that root end, make ½-inch slices through the head, one after another, cutting right down to the root. Discard the root, then place all those sliced bits in a colander set in the sink to rinse them of any grit under cool water.

Parmigiano-Reggiano is a hard, part-skim-milk cheese, originally from Italy but now made in the United States as well. Buy a chunk with the rind attached. There's no way you'll find exactly 2 ounces, so you'll get more than you need—which will be fine since we'll be using it quite a bit in the steps ahead. Seal it in plastic wrap and store it in the fridge. If you're paying for the real Italian deal, the cheese's name should be stamped on the rind. Look for pieces that are a pale creamy caramel without any desiccated bits along the edges.

MAKES 4 SERVINGS

S T E P

2

Make Informed Choices

WHAT WILL YOU DO?
Make chocolate pudding
Begin matching foods with elemental flavors
Learn how to make better choices

～～～～～～～～～

WHAT WILL YOU DISCOVER?
The incessant presence of fake food
The glory of herbs and spices
The real food chart

How to Be Faked Out

Let's start with pudding. Because it once was real food. And even easy to make. Just milk, eggs, sugar, a little flavoring, and perhaps a thickener like flour or cornstarch.

But that was before the onslaught of fake puddings, industrial-age wonders that remind us of the real thing. First came packaged mixes; next, instant puddings; then flip-top cans; and finally, shelf-stable snack packs. They're close enough, convenient enough, and cheap enough that many of us now mistake them for the real thing.[1]

To see what pudding had become after years of processing, Bruce and I bought four versions of these puddinglike conveniences. We opened or made each, lined them up on the kitchen counter, and did a taste test:[2]

BRAND	INGREDIENTS AS LISTED ON THE PACKAGE	DESCRIPTION	OUR THOUGHTS
ConAgra's Pudding Snacks, Chocolate Flavor	*Water, nonfat milk, sugar, modified cornstarch, vegetable oil (contains one or more of the following: palm oil, partially hydrogenated palm oil, sunflower oil, partially hydrogenated soybean oil), cocoa (processed with alkali), less than 2% of: salt, calcium carbonate, sodium stearoly lactate, artificial flavors, color added*	Fully made in a peel-open pack, no refrigeration required.	This shelf-stable product was quite smooth but had an oily texture and a rather bland taste, as if it were designed to offend the fewest people possible. It also had a depressingly chemical aftertaste and an unbelievably sweet cloyingness, nothing like real chocolate.

BRAND	INGREDIENTS AS LISTED ON THE PACKAGE	DESCRIPTION	OUR THOUGHTS
Jell-O Pudding Snacks, Chocolate Flavor	*Skim milk, sugar, modified food starch, cocoa processed with alkali, contains less than 1.5% of hydrogenated vegetable oil (coconut and palm kernel oils), cornstarch, salt, sodium stearoyl lactate (for smooth texture), sodium alginate, calcium phosphate, natural and artificial flavor, artificial color, vitamin A palmitate, vitamin D*	Fully made in a peel-open pack, but refrigeration is necessary.	The texture was hard to get over. It wasn't creamy but more like thick baby food: a little chewy (if that's a word for pudding) but also quite sticky. However, in fairness, the overall chocolate taste was the best of the four.
Jell-O Instant Pudding and Pie Filling, Chocolate Flavor	*Sugar, modified food starch, cocoa processed with alkali, disodium phosphate (for thickening), contains less than 2% of natural and artificial flavor, salt, tetra-sodium pyrophosphate (for thickening), mono- and dyglicerides (prevent foaming), red 40, yellow 5, blue 1, artificial color, BHA (preservative)*	A powdered, no-cook pudding mix that must be whisked into milk (we used low-fat), then chilled until set (3 minutes of whisking plus 15 minutes in the fridge).	This pudding had an unappealing plasticity and a livid sheen, quite dark, nearly black, with an unappealing chemical aftertaste. It required some minimal effort, but we wondered if that wasn't the point: to mimic cooking without actually being cooking.

BRAND	INGREDIENTS AS LISTED ON THE PACKAGE	DESCRIPTION	OUR THOUGHTS
My-T-Fine Pudding and Pie Filling, Chocolate Flavor	*Sugar, cornstarch, cocoa (processed with alkali), food starch (modified), contains less than 2% of the following: natural and artificial flavor, salt, partially hydrogenated soybean and cottonseed oil, calcium carrageenan (texturized), red 40, yellow 5, yellow 6, blue 1*	A powdered pudding made by whisking it into milk (again, we used low-fat) in a saucepan on the stove until bubbling, then chilling until set (14 minutes over the heat plus 30 minutes to set in the fridge).	This one tasted like chocolate the way a Tootsie Roll tastes like chocolate—as if it was supposed to remind us of chocolate. It was unpleasantly sweet, annoyingly so. The texture was smooth but strangely sticky. When we tried to pull a spoonful through our lips, the pudding stayed behind a bit, as if it were stuck to the flatware.

One phrase appeared on all the labels: *chocolate flavor*. Three of them called themselves that by name: not chocolate pudding, but *chocolate flavor pudding*. Indeed, they *were* doped with artificial flavor. (And color, too. Which got us to wondering, what color would they be without the fake coloring?)

However, the My-T-Fine brand did call itself simply *chocolate* (no *flavor* after the word).

Ah, we thought, *a real contender*.

Then we noticed that right under the word *chocolate* was emblazoned *artificial flavor added*. Were they proud of it?

Despite all this artificial flavor, every brand listed cocoa among its ingredients. Why would something made with cocoa powder (real food for sure) also need artificial flavor?

The cocoa, while of sufficient weight to get it listed fairly high in the ingredient ranks, might be of such poor quality that it contributes little to the pudding's overall flavor. Also, the chocolate flavor may need to be pumped up over and above any cocoa taste to cover the smack of the chemical residue. In other words, chemicals to the rescue of chemicals—although not enough. That metallic tang was hideously apparent in some versions.

But artificial flavors weren't the only chemicals. By our initial definition, pudding includes eggs. But there wasn't a yolk in our taste test. Not even powdered eggs, a processed substitute. Too bad, because egg proteins form the basic structure of pudding. In their loss, all the samples included a number of emulsifiers, thickeners, and stabilizers. That's apparently the game: lose one real thing and add a crazy number of fake things.

None of which adds up to real food. It's just chemical nostalgia: a processed fabrication that reminds us of a food we like.

Except all those additives aren't beside the point. And they aren't really *additives*, despite being so named. Instead, they make the concoction possible.

The Little Laboratory That Is Our Food

Once upon a time, the answers to modern life lay with these convenience products. They would give us more free time in an increasingly hyper world.

Unfortunately, speed comes at a chemical cost. Yes, artificial, manufactured, and processed additives have been developed so we can cook stuff more quickly. But then one thing leads to another. Other chemicals have to be added to make the now-doped products palatable again. Then still others have to be dumped inside to make the things last for weeks, months, and in some cases years. Do you really want to eat something that won't spoil until your birthday next year—or even the year after that?

There are more than three thousand so-called *additives* for foods sold in the United States.[3] They fall into three categories:

1. THOSE THAT ENHANCE NUTRITION

Mostly, these are vitamins, like the A added to milk. It's great that it's there: it's necessary for strong eyesight. However, it's found in (what should be) common foods: carrots, sweet potatoes, almost all leafy greens (like spinach), apricots, papayas, and mangos. Since we don't eat real food anymore, we have had to add essential nutrients where they don't naturally occur to make up for the deficit.

2. THOSE THAT INCREASE SHELF LIFE

Most are allegedly tasteless, designed to make sure the product doesn't absorb humidity or odors, doesn't mold, doesn't turn green, and doesn't do any number of things a piece of food naturally does when left out for months.

These additives are replacements for natural fats and proteins, all of which eventually go bad or rancid. So these particular additives extend the expiration dates. Think about it: we live in a world where food can *expire*—a term once used to indicate death, but now used to indicate a sell-by date for food made in a facility hundreds or even thousands of miles from our homes.

Are expiration dates a sign of fake food? Of course not. Milk, yogurt, and other dairy products do have a shelf life, even with proper storage. Expiration dates keep us safe. But we've come to a point where they're not a rarity on a handful of products. Rather, expiration dates are so common, they're barely noticed. They indicate a fundamental problem: shelf life has become more important than taste or nutrition.

Three of the most common additives are these:

Butilated Hydroxyanisole (BHA)
or Butilated Hydroxytoluene (BHT)
Organic compounds that preserve fats, keeping them from going rancid on the shelf. BHT is also used in jet fuel, exfoliating creams, and embalming fluids.

Erythorbic Acid and Sodium Erythorbate

A crystalline or granulated powder (the first is an acid and the second is a salt derived from it). Often made from beets or corn, it holds flavors stable over time—and increases shelf life by slowing down the formation of nitrosamines, known carcinogens in many preserved meats.

Sodium Benzoate

A granular salt that slows down the growth of bacteria and molds in acidic products including salad dressings, carbonated drinks, fruit juices, jams, and many condiments. It originated from a natural preservative found in plums, cranberries, and apples (benzoic acid) that does not dissolve very well and was thus reengineered for its life as a food additive. It's also the stuff that makes fireworks whistle.

3. THOSE THAT FAKE US OUT

Because of chemical additives, a soft drink can taste sweet without sugar. Mac-and-cheese can still be called mac-and-cheese without any real cheese. Cookies can taste buttery without real butter. And a chicken breast can taste like, well, chicken, without the bone, skin, or proper maturation in the barnyard.

Don't believe us? Check out the label on some of those packages of boneless, skinless breasts. It says they may contain up to 10 percent of a solution. . . . Then notice how the phrase trails off. Follow it down the packaging to discover that there's salt water injected into the meat as well as *artificial flavorings*. If they didn't add flavorings, what would the chicken breasts taste like?

Other food additives are more dangerous—like diacetyl, the chemical that gives a buttery flavor to items including microwave popcorn and hard candies. True, diacetyl adds no calories. That's its strong suit. It's also been linked to a life-threatening obstruction of lung passages, causing health alerts in factories where workers have been exposed to it. As of this writing, diacetyl is still considered safe by governmental agencies although it has been voluntarily re-moved by many manufacturers.

Then there's the depressing problem of chemical additives that have managed to become more real than the real thing itself. Benz-aldehyde replicates cherry flavor in candies, drinks, and desserts. But Robitussin is not cherry pie! Or maybe it is. The fake flavoring is now more recognizable to people as *cherry* than real cherries themselves.[4]

In fact, artificial flavorings are the big kahuna on the market. Of all the additives available today, almost half are flavoring agents, an incredible 500 percent growth since the fifties. By 1978, 80 percent of packaged and processed foods had some sort of flavor additive—and that was before the go-go eighties, the convenience nineties, or the mass hysteria of the millennial rush-rush.[5]

And all that is not to mention the emulsifiers (to keep fats and other things from falling out of suspension and forming an oily slick on a product), thickeners (to make things appear creamy when they can't be), texturizers (to make things feel better in the mouth than they in fact are), and gelling agents. Here's a sample of some of the most common food additives:

WHAT IT'S CALLED	WHAT IT IS	HOW IT'S USED
Calcium phosphate	A mineral, the basis of tooth enamel, and one of the major components in bones	A leavening agent, also used in commercial fertilizers
Calcium sulfate	Can be mined from gypsum	A common coagulant for tofu; when mixed with water, part of the formula for plaster of Paris
Carrageenan	A chemical compound extracted from seaweed	A gelling agent and thickener, keeps foods such as puddings homogenous

WHAT IT'S CALLED	WHAT IT IS	HOW IT'S USED
Cellulose gum	The most common thickening agent in processed foods, often made from the lints attached to cottonseeds	A texturizer (adds creamy mouthfeel), protein stabilizer, and a moisture retainer that forms an oil-resistant film in a huge range of foods from soups to condiments, from noodles to protein beverages
Dextrin, polydextrine, Maltodextrine	Processed short-chain starches	Low-calorie sweeteners and thickening agents
Dextrose, polydextrose	Forms of glucose (a.k.a. forms of sugar)	Low-calorie, lower-glucose sweeteners and thickeners added to salad dressings, low-calorie treats, and candies
Guar gum	Derivative of seeds from the guar plant, a legume	A thickener, often used in fat-free and low-fat products
Lecithin	A fatlike substance (a phospholipid), originally derived from egg yolks or milk but now extracted primarily from soy beans	An emulsifier, particularly able to keep fats in suspension, like the cocoa butter in chocolate
Locust bean gum	A processed gum from the endosperm of a leguminous carob tree	A stabilizer for gels and thickeners. It cannot gel on its own but improves the gel strength of other additives, particularly in the fillings for baked goods and canned pet food
Methylcellulose	A gummy substance that does not occur naturally	The primary component in digestive aids like Citrucel but also used as a thickener, absorbing humidity and water

WHAT IT'S CALLED	WHAT IT IS	HOW IT'S USED
Modified food starch, modified starch	Starches (corn, wheat, tapioca, etc.) heavily processed physically, chemically, and/or enzymatically to increase their stability against acids, heat, cold, or time	Thickeners, flow agents, antidrip agents in frozen foods, binders in low-fat meat products, the glue on postage stamps, and the goo in ultrasound liquids
Mono- and diglycerides	Modified fats, usually made from soybean, cottonseed, sunflower, or palm oil	Emulsifiers—both fat- and water-soluble. Thus, they join water and fat in an emulsion, keeping baked goods from getting stale
Polysorbate 20, 40, 60, 65, and 80	Oily liquids made when sorbitol (a sugar alcohol) is estrified with fatty acids	Texturizers that prevent proteins from coating fat droplets, allowing those proteins to create nets, thus allowing more air to get whipped into things and also providing a firmer texture (as something made with Polysorbate 80 melts, it retains its shape)
Sodium stearoyl lactylate and calcium stearoyl lactylate	A complex chemical compound made by combining lactic acid and stearic acid, then reacting the result with sodium hydroxide or calcium hydroxide	An emulsifier, particularly used in baked goods like tortillas or breads to keep them fresh
Tetrasodium pyrophosphate	Colorless, transparent crystals or a white powder	Stabilizer for acidity levels, binder of proteins to water (to hold together faux-crabmeat and chicken nuggets), and a thickener for instant puddings (also used in toothpaste to control tartar)
Xanthan gum	A residue produced when the bacteria are fed corn sugar	Thickener to give a creaminess to dressings, sauces, and desserts (also used to lubricate pumps)

What should we take away from all this information? In a world of expiring, shelf-stable, and fake-flavor foods, we ingest copious chemicals, metabolize them, store their residues in our cells, and convince ourselves that we're eating something real. Only to eat more because we're not. Which may be the biggest problem of all.

Full But Still Not Satisfied

Our brains process information, not nutrition. Regardless of whether our stomachs are getting the satisfaction they expect, if the chemical information in our food says *sweet* or *tasty* or *flavorful*, we chow down because our brains read taste first and foremost, based on memories of pleasure. Faked out, we then don't listen to what's going on down in our enteric nervous system.

For example, when we eat full-sugar, high-calorie foods, our brains sense the sweet, and all sorts of biochemical processes lurch into gear, preparing our bodies for lots of calories. Unfortunately, those very same processes come into play when we drink a diet soda. Our brains sense sweet—although fake—yet the real sugar never materializes. So our bodies are left waiting for calories. The artificial stuff has then broken the link between high-calorie foods and satiety. Faked out to expect more, we reach for more. And more.[6]

We've also trained ourselves to recognize the fake as the real. We've already seen the chocolate flavor in puddings. But what about fake vanilla, lemon, lime, cherry, watermelon, apple, orange, or banana? And nut flavors are often fake these days—or added to processed goods to enhance the taste of mealy, poor-quality nuts.

We've also let our brains fake out our stomachs when it comes to canned beef broth. It should be made with pan drippings—which are ridiculously expensive to produce on a mass scale. Therefore, many canned broths are stocked with monosodium glutamate (MSG), a chemical compound that we've now learned to interpret as *beef flavor*.

We've bought a bill of goods about how fake stuff is less fattening, less troublesome, less time-consuming, or just less costly—

when in fact it may be worse for us, more costly (in the long run), and to add insult to injury, more fattening.

But aren't all these additives safe? you might ask.

The short answer is *yes*.

But it's complicated.

There have been all sorts of investigative reports about additives—like the story of BHA and BHT. In 2007, the U.S. government ran tests and discovered that these two chemicals, long declared safe, can in fact react with vitamin C (ascorbic acid) or citric acid, added or naturally occurring in fruit and carbonated beverages. In the end, the lethal combo spawns benzene, a known carcinogen.

No one knows how much benzene we've imbibed over the years. Beverage manufacturers have since reformulated their products. Still, we have to wonder when the next shoe will fall.[7]

But let's be generous and give every additive in our food a bye. If we were resourceful, we could locate each one's original safety test. And we would find them cleared one by one. So is our short answer still *yes*?

Unfortunately, no.

Because no one has tested all those additives and preservatives for long-term use. They were given a human trial of forty days, three months, maybe a year, but not ten years, twenty years, thirty years, or more.

Except in us. We're *that* test. No one really knows what those chemicals or their broken-down residues do after years and years in our bodies, stored in the cellular structures we call ourselves.

And more tellingly, no one knows what those chemicals do in combination with each other, as with BHA or BHT and citric acid. Sure, a lab isolates an additive, tests it in rats, then humans, and finally releases it to the market. But what about that additive or preservative in combination with all the other chemicals we ingest? The residual antibiotics in our meat? The fertilizers in the animals' feed? And every drug we take? The statins? The aspirin? The antacids?

What about these little chemical experiments we call our bodies?

The First Solution: Real Chocolate Pudding

Enough with this house of horrors! The only escape is to go back to where we started: chocolate pudding. Nothing's more real or elemental. So make a batch and savor it. This version has an intense chocolate flavor, not sweet so much as satisfying, and a silky, luxurious texture.

2 large eggs

2 cups low-fat milk

⅓ cup packed light brown sugar

¼ cup cocoa powder

¼ cup unbleached all-purpose flour

1 ounce unsweetened or baking chocolate, hacked up into little bits

2 teaspoons vanilla extract

¼ teaspoon salt

1. Whisk the eggs in a large bowl. Give your forearm a workout to get the eggs smooth and creamy, without any floating bits of translucent egg white.

2. Put the milk, brown sugar, cocoa powder, flour, chocolate, vanilla, and salt in a large saucepan over medium heat and whisk until the chocolate melts and the mixture just begins to bubble. Cook, whisking while it bubbles lightly for 30 seconds.

3. Remove the pan from the heat and whisk half of this chocolate mixture into the eggs in a slow, steady stream until smooth. Whisk this combined mixture back into the remaining chocolate mixture in the saucepan, then set that pan over very low heat. If you're using an electric range, it may be helpful to use a second burner, just now turned to low. Whisk constantly over the heat for 2 minutes, reaching into the edges of the pan and letting the pudding come to only the barest bubble. If the pudding starts to bubble, reduce the heat even more or take the pan off the heat and keep whisking for a few seconds to cool it down.

4. Pour into four small ramekins or custard cups. Refrigerate until set, about 1 hour.

MAKES 4 SERVINGS

The Second Solution: Your Imagination

As you savor that chocolate pudding, imagine yourself as someone who relishes real food like this—someone who looks for it, understands why it's important, and won't settle for anything less.

What would it mean for your daily life? How would you approach dinner tonight? Would you put down the take-out menus to search for better options? Would you forget about making dinner out of half a box of crackers and some processed cheese spread?

This imaginative act is the framework of your future decisions. Hold it in your mind, a picture of who you can be.

The Third Solution: Take Your Glasses to the Grocery Store

To fulfill your vision, become a better shopper—which means you must become a better reader. All the information you need is on the cans, boxes, and packages. Bruce and I found it on the packages and containers of our chocolate puddings. In fact, all manufacturers are required to label what they make: to list the ingredients and nutritional information, among other things. Read those lists to find the fake-outs—and real food, too.

Take twenty minutes out of your day to make a trip to the grocery store, your glasses in hand if you need them. Don't shop; instead, stroll the aisles and look at the ingredients on random products. Read the labels on the frozen dinners, the cookies, even the stuff in the meat case. What's in that package of premarinated ribs? How many of those ingredients do you recognize? How many do you understand?

Be wary of any bursts or call-outs on the label: *High in Fiber! Sugar-Free! Fat-Free!* These often indicate that either something else is altered (it's high in fiber but also in sugar) or that a real food has been replaced with a fake substitute. *An important source of vitamin C* can simply mean the product is doped with sugars of all sorts—or even worse, that any real fruit has been replaced by chemical fake-outs and the C then added back for the health claim.

Yes, you'll find lots of processed crackers with chemical additives; but there are also others without any binders or emulsifiers. Right next to the processed chicken breasts with the chemical-laced marinades are real chicken breasts. Right next to the juices with artificial sweeteners and thickeners are the ones made from all juice.

You'll soon notice that one drawback to real food is its price. There are a few ways around this problem:

✦ Products go on sale occasionally. Stock up when you have the chance.

✦ Check out some Latin American, Mexican, or Chinese supermarkets. You'll be surprised at the low prices, particularly in the meat, dairy, and produce sections.

✦ Search out manufacturers' websites for coupons.

Not to make light of a very real problem, but the cost might help you value real food all the more.

The best news of all? You'll need less of better quality foods to feel more satisfied.

The Fourth Solution: More Flavor with Every Bite

Much of the fake stuff has been fabricated to put missing flavors into the chemical concoctions that have been passed off as real food. Since you've already become someone on the lookout for subtle flavor overtones, one way to resist the fake is to also relish big, bold flavors.

The best way to do that? Savor herbs and spices that bring lots of flavor to every bite. Use them in your cooking; find small restaurants where they are equally valued. Or go over the top and carry little bottles of dried oregano and chile powder with you!

Here's a handy chart to get you thinking about possible pairings for future meals:

WITH	USE
Chicken	Tarragon, basil, rosemary, thyme, oregano, ground cumin, ground fenugreek, ground ginger, paprika, and smoked paprika
Pork	Cilantro, rosemary, sage, thyme, oregano, fennel seeds, celery seeds, caraway seeds, red pepper flakes, grated nutmeg, ground cinnamon, cardamom, cloves, saffron, star anise
Beef	Sage, thyme, oregano, parsley, caraway seeds, celery seeds, smoked paprika, grated nutmeg, ground allspice, ground mace, ground cardamom
Fish	Anise, basil, lemon zest, oregano, savory, thyme, sage, ginger, fennel seeds, dill, chives
Leafy green vegetables	Red pepper flakes, ground cinnamon, ground allspice, grated nutmeg or mace
Tubers, roots, and hard vegetables	Mustard seeds, rosemary, oregano, thyme, red pepper flakes
Quick-cooking vegetables like broccoli or asparagus	Lemon zest, oregano, thyme, chervil, chives
Fruits	Thyme, lemon zest, ground cinnamon, star anise, freshly ground black pepper, crushed pink peppercorns

One note: relishing herbs and spices isn't automatic. None is preset in the brain. You have to learn their deep satisfaction by creating more memory tracks associated with pleasure.

Go to your spice rack or pantry, open the bottles of dried spices and herbs, and breathe in deeply. Get those flavors wired into your brain: nutmeg, cinnamon, tarragon, thyme, saffron, chile powder, oregano. Practice this every once in a while, just for a few minutes at a time. It'll help you become someone who savors and anticipates those very flavors. (And by the way, if a bottle doesn't smell like much, it's probably old and needs to be replaced. Dried herbs and spices can go bland after a year or so on the shelf.)

Here's a fun trip: find the nearest Penzey's, a spice purveyor with outlets across the country (to locate one, look at www .penzeys.com). At the store, you can sample hundreds of spices and blends. First, smell the simpler spices—like the several types of cinnamon. Then check out some of the bolder blends. Buy a few that you'd like to try. Now that's a lovely outing!

Now That We've Got You Thinking About Big, Bold Flavors . . .

No more chemical aftertaste! There's a goal. Try a couple of these recipes. All are heavy on the herbs and spices. Think about the flavors you've crafted in your meal. Set the table, pour yourself something to drink, and settle in.

TABBOULEH WITH SHRIMP, FETA, DILL, AND PARSLEY

Tabbouleh is traditionally a Middle Eastern salad made with bulgur wheat, mint, and tomatoes; here's a version Bruce has morphed to a main course with shrimp, feta, and two fresh herbs for more pleasure per bite. This dish is a great make-ahead for lunches or dinners; in fact, the flavors are best if they have a chance to mellow a bit. Cover the bowl with plastic wrap and store it in the refrigerator for up to three days.

1 cup quick-cooking bulgur wheat
(see Note)

1 cup boiling water

¼ pound medium shrimp (30 per
pound), peeled and deveined (see
Note, page 19)

2 large cucumbers, peeled, halved
lengthwise, any seeds scooped out
of the center, then the remaining
flesh cut into thin spears and diced
crosswise

Up to 1 small red onion, diced

1 cup chopped sun-dried tomatoes

½ cup crumbled feta (about 2 ounces)

⅓ cup packed parsley leaves, chopped

¼ cup lemon juice

2 tablespoons fresh dill, chopped, any
woody stems removed

2 tablespoons olive oil

½ teaspoon salt

½ teaspoon freshly ground black
pepper

1. Place the bulgur in a small bowl; stir in 1 cup boiling water. Cover and set aside for 30 minutes, until the water is absorbed and the bulgur is tender.

2. Meanwhile, bring a small saucepan of water to a boil over high heat. Add the shrimp and cook for about 2 minutes, just until pink and firm. Drain in a colander set in the sink, cool for a few minutes, then roughly chop the shrimp and place them in a medium serving bowl. If you want to avoid this step, look for precooked cocktail shrimp at the fish counter of your supermarket (you'll still need to chop them).

3. Fluff the bulgur with a fork, then add it to the shrimp.

4. Stir in the cucumber, red onion, sun-dried tomatoes, feta, parsley, lemon juice, dill, olive oil, salt, and pepper.

Note: In quick-cooking bulgur wheat, the kernels have been cleaned, parboiled, dried, and partially ground. Parboiling slightly reduces the fiber without reducing most of the nutrients.

MAKES 4 SERVINGS

MINESTRONE BURGERS

Veggie burgers are a go-to meal in our house: real food without much hassle. This version tastes like minestrone soup with some simple herbs and spices for good flavor. Serve the patties in whole wheat pita pockets with sliced tomatoes, crisp lettuce, and deli mustard. Or eat them on their own with a lightly dressed salad on the side. Or how about alongside Chilled Peach Soup (see pages 12–13)? The patties also make great leftovers—put a little olive oil in a skillet, set it over medium heat, and crisp the patties again, about two minutes per side.

¼ pound green beans

3 teaspoons olive oil, divided

½ cup red onion, chopped

2 medium garlic cloves, minced

1 large egg white

1¾ cups canned white beans, drained and rinsed

½ cup rolled oats (not quick-cooking or steel-cut oats)

2 teaspoons minced oregano leaves or 1 teaspoon dried oregano

2 teaspoons minced basil or 1 teaspoon dried basil

½ teaspoon red pepper flakes

½ teaspoon salt

½ cup sun-dried tomatoes, very finely chopped (see Note)

1. Bring a small saucepan of water to a boil over high heat. Add the green beans and cook for 1 minute. Drain in a colander set in the sink, then rinse with cool water until you can handle them. Chop into very small pieces, then set aside. If you want to avoid this whole step, chop thawed, frozen green beans without cooking them.

2. Heat 1 teaspoon of oil in a large skillet over medium heat. Add the onion and cook, stirring often, until somewhat soft, about 4 minutes. Add the garlic and cook for a few seconds, then pour the contents of the skillet into a food processor fitted with the chopping blade.

3. Add the egg white, beans, oats, oregano, basil, red pepper flakes, and salt. Process until smooth, scraping down the sides of the bowl as necessary.

4. Scrape the mixture into a large bowl; stir in the green beans and sun-dried tomatoes.

5. Heat the remaining 2 teaspoons oil in that large skillet over medium heat. Scoop up ½ cup of the mixture and form it into a patty. It will be sticky, so make a loose, slightly irregular patty. If you wet your hands before digging into it, the whole operation goes better. Set that patty in the skillet and continue making more, as many as will fit comfortably. Cook for 4 minutes, then flip and continue cooking for 4 more minutes, until brown and crisp. If you can't fit them all in the skillet, you'll need to add 2 more teaspoons of oil for the second batch.

Note: Look for pliable, soft sun-dried tomatoes, not those soaked in oil but instead the dry ones that are among the other produce at your supermarket. If they're particularly hard and unyielding, pour boiling water over them in a small bowl and soak for 10 minutes before draining and chopping.

MAKES 6 PATTIES

POACHED SALMON WITH DILL-CUCUMBER SAUCE

This herbed-up, no-cook sauce is modeled on tzatziki, a traditional Greek preparation. Want to make this dish for a dinner party some weekend? Double the amounts, using a 2½- to 3-pound salmon fillet.

1½ cups dry white wine or dry
    vermouth (see Notes, page 28)
1½ cups water
1 medium shallot, minced
4 bay leaves
4 whole cloves
1¼ to 1½ pounds skin-on salmon fillet
1 small cucumber

½ cup Greek-style yogurt
1 tablespoon lemon juice
1 tablespoon minced dill fronds or
    1½ teaspoons dried dill
1 teaspoon honey
½ teaspoon dry mustard
¼ teaspoon salt
¼ teaspoon freshly ground black pepper

1. Bring the wine or vermouth, water, shallot, bay leaves, and cloves to a simmer in a high-sided skillet or sauté pan large enough to hold the piece of salmon.

2. Ease the fillet into the skillet or pan. Bring the liquid back to a simmer; then cover, reduce the heat to very low, and simmer slowly for 2 minutes. Turn off the heat and set the covered pan aside on another, cool burner for 15 minutes.

3. Meanwhile, peel the cucumber, then cut it in half lengthwise. Use a small spoon to scrape out and discard the seeds. Slice each of the halves lengthwise into thin strips, then slice these crosswise into a thin dice.

4. Mix the cucumber pieces, yogurt, lemon juice, dill, honey, dry mustard, salt, and pepper in a medium bowl.

5. After the salmon has steeped for 15 minutes, gently transfer the fillet to a cutting board. You'll need two flat spatulas and some deft coordination. Discard the liquid and all the aromatics. Slice the salmon crossways (not lengthwise) into four servings. Transfer these to serving plates and spoon the yogurt sauce over them.

MAKES 4 SERVINGS

VEGETABLE BIRYANI

Now things get a little more complicated. Some spice mixtures come preprepared, such as garam masala, which means *warm spice*—in other words, not fiery but comforting. There are hundreds of various blends available from gourmet supermarkets, East Indian supermarkets, or online suppliers. To serve this classic casserole, either scoop it onto plates with a big spoon or take the more traditional approach: turn the baking dish upside down onto a large serving platter, dumping out the casserole to be scooped up by those at the table. Serve it with some jarred chutney (see page 228), minced chives, and/or chopped cilantro leaves for garnishes.

½ cup long-grain brown rice, such as brown jasmine or brown basmati rice

1¼ cups water

1 tablespoon sesame oil

1 small yellow onion, chopped

1 medium tomato, chopped

1 medium garlic clove, chopped

1 tablespoon minced peeled fresh ginger or jarred chopped ginger

6 cups mixed vegetables such as small cauliflower florets (or larger ones cut into small pieces), small broccoli florets (or larger florets cut into smaller pieces), green beans (cut into 1-inch pieces), frozen peas, carrots, thinly sliced, and yellow squash or zucchini, diced

1½ tablespoons garam masala (see Note)

1 teaspoon ground cinnamon

½ teaspoon salt

¼ cup plain regular or low-fat yogurt

1 tablespoon lemon juice

¼ cup almonds, walnuts, or pecans, chopped

¼ cup raisins, preferably golden raisins, chopped

1 tablespoon unsalted butter, melted, if desired

1. Mix the rice and water in a medium pot; bring to a simmer over medium-high heat, stirring occasionally. Cover the pot, reduce the heat to very low, and simmer slowly until the rice is tender, 30 to 40 minutes. Set the pot aside, off the heat, while you prepare the casserole.

2. Position a rack in the center of the oven and preheat to 350°F.

3. Heat a large saucepan over medium heat. Add the sesame oil, then add the onion, tomato, garlic, and ginger. Cook until the onion has begun to soften and the tomatoes to break down, about 5 minutes, stirring once in a while.

4. Stir in the vegetables, garam masala, cinnamon, and salt. Stir over the heat until quite aromatic, about 2 minutes.

5. Stir in the yogurt and lemon juice. Cover the pot, reduce the heat to low, and simmer slowly until the vegetables have begun to break down, about 20 minutes, stirring once in a while.

6. Stir in the nuts and raisins and set the pot aside, off the heat.

7. Spread half the rice in the bottom of a 9-inch square baking dish. Pour all the vegetable mixture on top; spread it evenly to the cor-

ners. Top the dish with the remaining rice, again spreading it evenly across the baking dish.

8. Cover with aluminum foil and bake for 15 minutes. Let stand at room temperature, covered, for 5 minutes. If desired, preheat the broiler and place the rack about 6 inches from the heat source. Brush the melted butter over the casserole, then set it under the broiler just until the rice begins to get a little crisp. Set the casserole aside at room temperature for 5 minutes before turning the whole thing upside down onto a large serving platter.

Note: If you want to take your spice knowledge to higher levels, consider making your own garam masala. In any quantities, mix together 1 part ground allspice, 1 part cayenne, 2 parts fennel seeds, 4 parts mild paprika, 4 parts ground cumin, 4 parts ground cardamom, and 8 parts ground coriander. For example, use ½ teaspoon as 1 part—then take it from there. You'll make more than you need, but you can store the mixture in the spice cabinet for up to 9 months, using it on scrambled eggs, in mac-and-cheese, or as a garnish on steamed or roasted vegetables.

MAKES 4 SERVINGS

(CAN BE DOUBLED IF PUT INTO A 9 X 13-INCH BAKING DISH)

DRIED APRICOT AND CHICKEN TAGINE

A tagine is a long-stewed Moroccan casserole, a spice extravaganza. It's usually made in a specialty pot, but Bruce's version is simpified for the equiptment most of us have. His version is also quicker and fresher, thanks to the bright spike of dried California apricots, which are orange and tart. (Dried Turkish apricots tend to be milder in flavor and have less juice per bite.) Consider this an advanced recipe in your quest for more flavor through herbs and spices.

1 tablespoon olive oil

2 medium yellow onions, thinly sliced

4 medium garlic cloves, slivered

1 tablespoon minced peeled fresh
    ginger or jarred preminced ginger

2 pounds boneless, skinless chicken
    thighs, cut into 2-inch pieces

1 teaspoon ground cinnamon

1 teaspoon ground coriander

1 teaspoon ground cumin

½ teaspoon salt

½ teaspoon freshly ground black
    pepper

¼ teaspoon ground cloves

2 cups reduced-sodium vegetable
    broth

1²/₃ cups canned chickpeas, drained
    and rinsed

1 cup dried California apricots,
    chopped

1 tablespoon honey

One 9-ounce box frozen baby
    artichokes, thawed and gently
    squeezed in batches over the sink
    to remove most of the excess
    moisture without smooshing them

1. Preheat the oven to 375°F. Heat the oil in a large flame-safe casserole or Dutch oven over medium heat. Add the onion; cook, stirring often, until softened, about 4 minutes.

2. Add the garlic and ginger; cook for 1 minute, stirring constantly.

3. Add the chicken; cook, stirring often, until lightly browned, about 4 minutes.

4. Stir in the cinnamon, coriander, cumin, salt, pepper, and cloves; cook until aromatic, about 20 seconds.

5. Pour in the broth; scrape up any browned bits on the pan's bottom. Stir in the chickpeas, dried apricots, and honey. Bring to a simmer; then cover, place in the oven, and bake for 45 minutes.

6. Sprinkle the artichoke bits over the casserole without stirring them in. Cover and continue baking until bubbling and thick, about 15 more minutes. Set aside, covered, at room temperature for 10 minutes before stirring and serving.

MAKES 6 SERVINGS

Keeping It Real

Once Bruce and I decided to forget fake food and make real food our goal, we made this quick inventory of our fridge:

✦ On the top shelf: containers of milk and yogurt in various fat percents, as well as a couple sticks of butter and a carton of eggs.

✦ On the main shelves, the vast bulk of the food: some leftover pasta salad from recipe-testing for a magazine article, a doggy bag with pieces of roast chicken from a restaurant, bits of a pork roast and vegetables from a dinner party, plus containers of dips, plastic-wrapped bits of cheese, deli meats, and a box of crackers. (How did those get in there?)

✦ On the door shelves: sun-dried tomatoes and stuffed grape leaves from the supermarket's salad bar, as well as jars or bottles of jam, mustard, salad dressing, oil, hot fudge sauce, barbecue sauce, salsa, hot sauce, and mayonnaise.

✦ In the hydrators: chicken thighs and beef bottom round for recipe-testing, a few navel oranges, a pear and some celery ribs that had seen better days, two heads of cauliflower (two?), and a bag of onions.

✦ Scattered all around, the snacks: applesauce, peanut butter, raspberries from a local farm, and the remnants of a strawberry-rhubarb crisp from that same dinner party. Plus, a half-eaten candy bar. (Don't even ask.)

And that's not counting what was in the freezer. (Butter-pecan ice cream, anyone?) With so much on hand, how could we know what was real food? Those condiments? The yogurt? That half-eaten candy bar? How could we choose?

The Real Food Chart

In truth, what was in our refrigerator did not fall into neat categories of real and fake food. It was far more complicated. We needed a forgiving and flexible system for reference.

Here's what we finally came to: there's the best of all possible foods, some great substitutes, some barely acceptable ones, and a host of things that aren't real food in any sense of the word. Therefore, our system goes like this:

REAL FOOD	ALMOST REAL FOOD	BARELY REAL FOOD	NOT REAL FOOD

Let's take the boxes one by one.

REAL FOOD

This category includes fruits, vegetables, beans, berries, meat, fish, shellfish, eggs, whole grains, spices, herbs, nut oils, olive oil, milk, cream, and even butter. The majority of the things in this box are basic ingredients from the grocery store—or solid preparations (like those recipes for tabbouleh or biryani) that emphasize the satisfying, natural, fresh taste of their real ingredients.

In our homemade chocolate pudding, for example, most of the ingredients were as close to their natural state as possible.[8] We made a chocolate pudding that actually included chocolate and that actually tasted like chocolate. "An adult pudding," one of our recipe testers called it.

So real food is not only the elemental ingredients; it also offers a full range of fats, sugars, fiber, and protein. In fact, real food leads to greater pleasure and satiety precisely because it encompasses this range. Real food is steak and potatoes, bread and chocolate.

Take broccoli, that most dreaded of all vegetables. Forget a boiled mess of flabby green. How about broccoli stir-fried in sesame oil with chiles and scallions for a tongue-spanking pop? Or cooked in a skillet with walnut oil and sliced onions for a beat-back-winter freshness? Or roasted with olive oil, grated lemon zest, and whole garlic cloves so the natural sugars mingle and caramelize?

That all said, it's still real food if the prep work has been done for you—for example, prechopped butternut squash from the supermarket's produce section or cut-up vegetables for a stir-fry. Even the salmon burgers at the supermarket can be real food, although they're premade and preformed. The time you spend preparing something is no indicator of whether it counts as real food. Convenience should never be discounted, just examined.

In the end, real foods retain their nutritional goodness and flavors by using honest, real ingredients without resorting to chemicals and fakes.

However, some processing retains and even enhances a food's natural character. Boiling down maple sap to make maple syrup? Perfectly acceptable. Drying herbs to make bottled spices? Terrific. Crushing olives into oil or milling grains into flours? Fully real food. Churning cream into butter? Who could live without it?

Or take chocolate. Few of us would eat a cacao bean off the tree. To turn the beans into chocolate, they're dried, fermented, ground, then mixed with sugars and more cocoa fat. But no one would doubt that chocolate is real food because (1) all that processing creates a product amazingly in line with the pods off the tree, and (2) nothing chemical *has to be added* to the cocoa beans along the way.

In like manner, coffee and tea are real foods because even if you got the beans or leaves home, you'd have to complete the same process as manufacturers to turn them into something you can drink.

However, if the processing removes essential flavors, chances are the product is no longer real food. For example, refining often takes away most of a vegetable oil's taste, robbing us of what we need in order to know we're full. Rather than a tasteless oil, how about a full-flavored walnut or avocado oil?

Here's another example. Cocoa butter is often chemically deodorized to make white chocolate, robbing it of any cocoa taste.

Even worse are versions of so-called white chocolate that are no more than hydrogenated shortening with fake flavorings. Better then to find a true white chocolate, with the trace flavors of the darker cocoa still in place.

If the processing transforms something good into something bad for you—like vegetable fats that get hydrogenated into solid shortenings (more on this in "Step 4")—it's not real food anymore.

Or if the processing robs the food of a high percentage of its nutritional value, it's probably not real food.

But real food is not necessarily raw. Real food can be cooked to retain its natural goodness. And it's not simply old-fashioned. There was a food-lover's rule a while back that basically said you should eat things only your grandparents or great-grandparents would recognize as food. Unfortunately, that's too simplistic. After all, shrimp was bait until the late-nineteenth century.

Remember that real food is about getting back to two important standards: taste and health.

ALMOST REAL FOOD AND BARELY REAL FOOD

Of course, not all foods can fall into the first box on the left of our chart. So we have two categories just to the right of the ideal: *almost real food* and *barely real food*. As we go along, we'll fill in these boxes with foods and products based on the amount of processing, added fat or sugar, chemicals, or a few other dietary concerns.

For example, while a fresh peach remains our goal, we don't live in a perfect world. Deep in December, we can only get the little hard golf balls from Chile. We might then put those in that box to the right, *almost real food*, something we have to use because there are few other choices at that time of year.

Or we might even put frozen sliced peaches in that category. No, they're not good for eating on their own, but they can be used in our Chilled Peach Soup (see pages 12–13) to good effect.

Think back to those pears we tried from the can. The ones doped with too much sugar would fall one box farther over, into *barely real food*. As long as they're not laced with artificial junk, they're still within the realm of the real; but they're really not a good choice, given their slimy, overly sweet taste.

In fact, many canned products would end up in one of these two categories. Remember: we've got two key criteria—taste and health. So canned beans—just like high-quality, organic canned broth and jarred artichoke hearts or roasted red peppers packed in water— would fall into the *almost real food* box because (1) they retain a good portion of their fiber and nutrients, and (2) they taste pretty good, close to the real food you would make yourself. Besides, canned beans are a terrific time-saver. So a soup made with them would be *almost real food*—and definitely good enough to make the cut.

That said, canned bean soup may contain too many preservatives and chemicals. It then would fall farther to the right on our chart and into the danger zone. Which is . . .

NOT REAL FOOD

These are foods and ingredients doped with additives, laced with artificial flavors, and/or thickened chemically. They include a host of packaged, processed, and convenience products.

And horrifyingly, they include most of the fruit we eat— because we don't eat real fruit anymore! By 1998, 56 percent of all fruit consumed in the United States was processed into spreads, doughnut fillings, pie fillings, and other convenience products.[9] Whatever happened to just eating a piece of fruit?

Many frozen peach pies would also end up in this last box because of the sheer size of their chemical signature. However, some would escape, becoming *barely real food*. And a homemade peach pie, made with sliced fresh peaches and a buttery crust would certainly fall in *almost real food*, if not *real food* altogether, depending on the ingredients used.

Fat-free half-and-half is *not real food*. How do you know? Read the label: thickeners aplenty and corn syrup sweeteners. Here's the listed ingredients on one brand: *Nonfat Milk, Corn Syrup, Cream, Artificial Color, Sodium Citrate, Dipotassium Phosphate, Mono- &*

Diglycerides, Carrageenan, Vitamin A Palmitate. Something consummately real has been turned into fake food in short order—although there is somehow cream in the fat-free version. Talk about bizarre! Here's something that is itself and isn't.

Okay, so let's begin to build a full chart. Why not just enjoy real half-and-half? In moderation, of course.

REAL FOOD	ALMOST REAL FOOD	BARELY REAL FOOD	NOT REAL FOOD
Freshly squeezed orange juice	Orange juice not from concentrate	Orange juice from concentrate	Bottled orange-flavored drink
An apple, nothing-added applesauce, dried apple rings, or unsweetened apple cider	Sweetened applesauce (without any fake stuff)	Fake-flavored applesauce	Sugar-free canned apple pie filling
An apricot, dried apricots without preservatives	Frozen apricot halves, apricots canned in juice (without any artificial sweeteners)	Canned apricots in light syrup	Artificially sweetened canned apricots and apricot-flavored juice drinks
A tomato, fragrant or pliable sun-dried tomatoes	Natural, salt-free canned tomatoes or pliable, fragrant sun-dried tomatoes	Preflavored, salted, stewed tomatoes; and sun-dried tomatoes packed in oil with added flavorings	Condensed tomato soup, most bottled ketchup
Fresh artichokes	Frozen artichoke hearts	Canned artichoke hearts	Prebreaded, prefried, preseasoned frozen artichoke hearts; many canned artichoke dips
A potato, baked, roasted, boiled, mashed, steamed, or oven-fried	Premade (fresh or frozen) natural, mashed potatoes; all natural frozen potato and vegetable blends	Frozen fried potatoes	Tater Tots, instant mashed potatoes, canned potato strings

REAL FOOD	ALMOST REAL FOOD	BARELY REAL FOOD	NOT REAL FOOD
Nondeodorized, artisanal white chocolate made from cocoa butter	None	Run-of-the-mill white chocolate	White chocolate made with fats other than cocoa butter
Fresh mozzarella	A block of shrink-wrapped mozzarella	String-style, low-moisture, part-skim mozzarella	Frozen, breaded, prefried mozzarella sticks
Fresh pasta	Dried pasta	Frozen, cooked pasta (depending on the sauce, it may slip one category to the right)	Canned pasta
Whole grains, like wheat berries or oats	Whole wheat bread and whole-grain breakfast cereals	Whole wheat bread doped with corn syrup	Processed white sandwich bread or processed frozen rolls; most of the breads or rolls that come out of a can
A fresh or smoked ham, including in-store roasted ham from the store's deli	Packaged, cooked whole hams without chemicals or additives	Presliced deli ham (especially if loaded with nitrates or other chemicals)	Canned ham under a key, canned deviled ham, shrink-wrapped ham salad
Bone-in chicken parts	Boneless skinless chicken parts	Canned chicken	Frozen, prebreaded chicken nuggets

Hold this chart in your mind. Make your own version, if you want. Put it in your briefcase or purse. As you go about your day, think about what's real and what's not, what's almost real food and what's barely so, what's been shellacked with additives, what's wonderful in its natural state.

Test Case 1: Mandarin Oranges

Canned mandarin oranges once ruled grocery store shelves—mostly because nobody could find a fresh one. Originally from Asia, it's a small orange, perfumed like a tangerine, but a little sweeter and without the vanilla overtones.

These days, many of us can buy fresh mandarins in the late winter. However, canned versions remain the dominant way we experience this fruit: tossed into the Asian salads at many chain restaurants, added to stir-fries in some Chinese restaurants, or even suspended in our great aunt's Jell-O salad.

As an experiment, Bruce and I set out to discover how various versions of a mandarin orange would fit into our real food chart. We used:

✦ a fresh mandarin orange

✦ no-sugar-added canned mandarin orange sections packed in water

✦ canned mandarin orange sections packed in juice (in pear juice, to be exact)

✦ canned mandarin orange sections packed in light syrup

The fresh mandarin orange scored as *real food*, no problem; so we set it in that category without any qualms.

Then things got trickier. When we sat down to examine our options, we believed the orange sections packed in light syrup would merit our greatest scorn. How could these be real food with that overly sweet, sticky shellac?

And let's not kid ourselves: they were sweet, overwhelmingly so, almost enough to mask the natural flavors.

But here's where it got complicated: we were equally shocked at the sections packed in water. They, too, were very sweet, unexpectedly so. In fact, they tasted sweeter than those packed in the light syrup. What was up?

The label blared *no sugar added*. A good sign, we thought. Then we noted a little symbol at the bottom of the can. A footnote, as it were. We put on our reading glasses.

Although there was no sugar added, there was Splenda. And when we read the ingredients on the back, we discovered that these mandarin sections were doped three times over with chemical sweeteners: with sorbitol, acesulfame potassium, and sucralose. What appeared to be a healthful choice was actually laced with fake stuff. How did we know? By reading the can's federally mandated ingredient list on the back, not by paying attention to the labeling tricks on the front.

While we're on the subject, what were the ingredients in our canned selections? Here they are, exactly as listed on the labels:

✦ no-sugar-added canned mandarin orange sections packed in water: *mandarin oranges, water, sorbitol, citric acid, artificial sweeteners (acesulfame potassium, sucralose), cellulose gum*

✦ canned mandarin orange sections packed in juice: *mandarin orange segments, pear juice*

✦ canned mandarin orange sections packed in light syrup: *mandarin orange segments, water, sugar, citric acid*

Two of our selections included citric acid—which has two purposes in modern processed foods. It's a preservative and it also gives a sour pop. The white powdery stuff on sour candies is often citric acid. It's probably added here to keep the orange sections in good shape and also give back a little of the sour spark they've lost in processing.

Then there's that cellulose gum (see page 39), added to make the sections slipperier, a little chewier. Perhaps the water-packed segments are trying to mimic the ones packed in syrup, a little slick chewiness in each bite?

In the end, the sections packed in *light syrup* had fewer fake-out chemicals than the *no sugar added* ones. So gathering all our information, here's our chart:

REAL FOOD	ALMOST REAL FOOD	BARELY REAL FOOD	NOT REAL FOOD
Fresh mandarin segments	Mandarin orange sections in pear juice	Mandarin orange sections in light syrup	No-sugar-added mandarin orange sections in water (artificially sweetened)

Do you need to do this sort of over-the-top investigation at every step? Of course not. But open your eyes to the possibilities and the limits of your choices.

Left to our own assumptions, Bruce and I would have put the canned oranges in light syrup down at the bottom as *not real food*. But by reading labels and ingredient lists, we were able to better see how our choices fell out—and make better ones at that.

Two More Examples Along the Lines of Those Mandarin Oranges

A significant number of processed products have been born out of convenience, to mimic what we can make at home. Are they all bad? By no means! Just as we did with our mandarin oranges, we have to do a little investigating.

In other words, we have to take our glasses to the supermarket. Or put another way, we have to treat a supermarket like a bookstore, as if it were stocked with things to read (as well as to eat). Will doing so slow us down? Yes, a bit. But the payoff will be beyond compare: we will become the kind of people who accept nothing less than the best. We don't just seek convenience (although we don't discount it either); we instead seek satisfaction at all times.

Two of the most common convenience products are pasta sauces and salad dressings. How do these things fit into our chart?

REAL FOOD	ALMOST REAL FOOD	BARELY REAL FOOD	NOT REAL FOOD
A pot of homemade marinara sauce (made from fresh or canned tomatoes—as long as the can has no chemical additives). Or a jarred marinara sauce made from real ingredients like tomatoes, onions, green pepper, olive oil, salt, and herbs. Tomatoes should be the first ingredient in the list (not tomato paste or any reconstituted tomato product) and there should be no artificial colors, flavors, thickeners, or other additives	A jarred marinara sauce made from real ingredients, i.e., tomatoes, onions, green pepper, olive oil, salt, and herbs. However, there may be some stretchers in the mix (most likely, water) or perhaps some sort of tasteless fat. There may also be citric acid to increase zip and freshness	A jarred marinara sauce made with some sort of processed tomato product (puree, paste, etc.) with some sugar in the mix (which just indicates that the tomatoes were of inferior quality, weren't sweet enough on their own), as well as some dehydrated vegetables (onions, garlic)	A jarred marinara sauce stocked with thickeners, preservatives, flavoring additives, corn syrup, and emulsifiers
A homemade or bottled salad dressing whisked together from a flavorful oil (like olive oil), a flavorful acid (like white wine vinegar or lemon juice), and some herbs or spices— or one from real mayonnaise (no artificial stabilizers or thickeners), buttermilk, or sour cream with only natural flavorings and real ingredients	A homemade or bottled salad dressing made with a tasteless oil (like *salad oil*—more on this in "Step 4"), but other real ingredients, and perhaps citric acid or a sodium derivative thrown in to preserve freshness	A bottled salad dressing made with a flavorless oil, stocked with dehydrated dairy products or herbs, as well as sugar or corn syrup	A chemically charged bottled product with artificial sweeteners, artificial flavors and colors, guar gum and a host of thickeners, as well as tasteless oil and run-of-the-mill vinegar

We could make the same categorizations with soup (from home-made to various canned versions), whipped cream (from the canned stuff that's just real cream with a propellant, to the chocolate versions with fake flavors, to the all-fake stuff), and even bread (from crunchy baguettes made only with flour, water, yeast, and salt, to gummy, presliced breads stocked with sweeteners and preservatives, an enormous chemical signature).

Although the first category, *real food*, is what we strive for, we cannot achieve it at every turn. Life needs more forgiveness. Therefore, the two categories to its right, *almost real food* and *barely real food*, are ways to get close enough, especially at the beginning of this journey. By the end, we hope to choose only items in the first two categories. For now, keep this in mind: whatever you've been doing, however you've been buying food, strive to move your choices one category to the left. If you find that most of what you've got or buy is *barely real food*, then make it your goal to start shopping for things that would fall into the *almost real food* category—better pasta, better salad dressings.

And speaking of those, here are some *real food* versions to get you started:

NO-COOK TOMATO PASTA SAUCE

This sauce is best when tomatoes are at their peak in midsummer. It can be saved in the fridge for a day or two but let it come back to room temperature before tossing it with still-warm whole wheat spaghetti.

6 tablespoons olive oil
½ teaspoon white wine vinegar
¼ teaspoon sugar
¼ teaspoon salt

¼ teaspoon freshly ground black
   pepper
2 pounds ripe Italian or plum
   tomatoes (4 to 5 large tomatoes)
¼ cup basil leaves, chopped

1. Whisk the oil, vinegar, sugar, salt, and pepper in a large bowl.

2. Cut the tomatoes into several sections, then hold these over the sink or a trash can and scoop out the seeds and their membranes with a small spoon or your finger.

3. Finely chop the seeded tomatoes. Stir them and the basil into the olive oil dressing.

MAKES 4 SERVINGS

MARINARA

This may be the most versatile pasta sauce, a simple taste that beats any jarred version. Serve it over just about any pasta shape you choose—so long as you also give it a good sprinkle of real finely grated Parmigiano-Reggiano on top.

2 tablespoons olive oil

1 medium onion, finely chopped

2 or 3 medium garlic cloves, minced

1 tablespoon minced oregano or
    2 teaspoons dried oregano

1 tablespoon stemmed thyme or
    2 teaspoons dried thyme

3½ cups canned reduced-sodium diced
    tomatoes

1 bay leaf

¼ teaspoon grated nutmeg

¼ teaspoon salt

¼ teaspoon freshly ground black
    pepper

1. Heat a medium saucepan over medium heat. Pour in the oil, add the onion, and cook until soft, about 3 minutes, stirring frequently.

2. Add the garlic, oregano, and thyme; cook just until you can smell the herbs, about 10 seconds.

3. Pour in the tomatoes, stir in the bay leaf and nutmeg, then bring to a simmer.

4. Reduce the heat to low, simmer uncovered until somewhat thickened, not soupy at all, about 25 minutes. Season with salt and pepper. Remove and discard the bay leaf before serving.

MAKES 4 SERVINGS

ASIAN PEANUT DRESSING

Leave behind the majority of bottled salad dressings; most are full of fake flavorings and tasteless fats. This one's a version of that sweet and savory dressing served over the salad at many Japanese restaurants. Try it over any shredded radishes, carrots, celery root, or zucchini (or a mixture of any two). Or just put it on some chopped Romaine lettuce for an easy side salad.

6 tablespoons peanut oil

¼ cup rice vinegar (see Note, page 114)

1 tablespoon creamy natural peanut
   butter

1 tablespoon soy sauce

1 teaspoon dried ginger

Whisk all the ingredients in a small bowl until smooth. The dressing can be saved in the fridge for up to 3 days, whisking it again to thin it out before using.

MAKES SIX 2-TABLESPOON SERVINGS

HONEY-MUSTARD VINAIGRETTE

This dressing is best on a composed salad: some chopped lettuce, a sliced peach or plum, a few chopped nuts or crumbled goat cheese, some radish sprouts, and precooked cocktail shrimp.

6 tablespoons olive oil or walnut oil

¼ cup white wine vinegar

1 tablespoon Dijon mustard

2 teaspoons honey

1 garlic clove, mashed

½ teaspoon freshly ground black
   pepper

¼ teaspoon salt

Whisk all the ingredients in a small bowl. The dressing can be made ahead of time and kept at room temperature for up to 6 hours—or in the fridge for up to 3 days.

MAKES SIX 2-TABLESPOON SERVINGS

Test Case 2: Fried Fish

One weekend, Bruce and I went to our friends' house for dinner. The adults had a lovely meal: roast turkey, steamed butternut squash, broccoli. Even an apple pie for dessert. But the kids had none of it. They had fish sticks, scraped off a baking sheet, plopped down in a pile of ketchup.

We're not unsympathetic. Our friends work demanding jobs. They had company to entertain and were just trying to keep the peace. But on the way home, Bruce and I thought about those ever-present fish sticks, a go-to meal for kids (and adults, too). Where do they fall in our chart?

Without a doubt, the fish stick arises from the healthiest way to fry fish, a technique called oven-frying: fish fillets are lightly coated and set on a baking sheet in a hot oven until crunchy. No excess oil, no overly fatty coating—*if* you make it yourself. However, the pre-breaded ones in the supermarket's freezer section have a high-fat coating, made with all sorts of tasteless binders and preservatives. Plus, the fish is processed, chopped, and probably extruded, sort of like fish mush.

Bruce and I did posit that there was probably an alternative: organic, low-processed fish fillets at high-end supermarkets. We hadn't seen them but thought they must exist. We figured our chart would look like this:

REAL FOOD	ALMOST REAL FOOD	BARELY REAL FOOD	NOT REAL FOOD
Oven-fried fish fillets	Organic oven-fried fish fillets	None really	Processed, frozen, prebreaded, preformed fish fillets

It seemed straightforward. But my hunch was that few people would ever bother to make their own oven-fried fish fillets. I did a random sampling among our friends. "If you know oven-fried fish fillets are better for you and more satisfying," I asked them, "why do you ever make the frozen, packaged stuff?"

Time and again, I ran into two answers: cost and time.

I bought the answers at face value, so much so that one day I brought up my little survey with a food-writer friend and ended up in a rather heated argument. I argued that real food was more costly than the fake—and that not everyone could make the choice for real food so easily.

He scoffed at me. "You've just bought the marketing gimmicks of the processed-food makers."

I was duly outraged. But it turns out, I had.

Bruce set up a taste test between our own version of oven-fried fish and a store-brand competitor of frozen, breaded fish fillets. Here's what we thought we'd discover: that the store-bought fillets were cheaper and quicker, but ours tasted better. (Hey, no point in hiding our prejudices.)

So he upped the ante. He added a premium version of those breaded fillets to give ours a run for their money, those great substitutes we'd theorized existed. He drove to a high-end supermarket to find sustainable, line-caught, whole wheat–breaded frozen fish. Unfortunately, they had no fillets, but they did have some premium fish sticks made from sliced, whole cod fillets.

He also bought the fresh fish fillets from that same market. The haddock looked particularly fresh, but frankly just about any thin, white-fleshed fish fillet would have worked.

He got it all home and set to cooking. We timed the preparation and figured out the cost and calories. Based on the serving sizes on the packaging, here are our results:

	REAL FOOD: OUR HOMEMADE OVEN-FRIED HADDOCK FILLETS	ALMOST REAL FOOD: NATURAL SEA PREMIUM COD FISH STICKS	NOT REAL FOOD: STOP & SHOP CRUNCHY FISH FILLETS
Serving size[10]	106 g (3.73 ounces)	106 g (3.73 ounces)	108 g (3.81 ounces)
Time spent to prepare	28 minutes	19 minutes	24 minutes
Cost	$1.11	$3.20	$1.30
Calories	180	221	290

Not only were our fillets lower in calories than the other two, they were also cheaper. Admittedly, ours weren't as quick. They took four minutes longer than the Stop & Shop fillets and nine minutes more than the Natural Sea sticks. But it wasn't *that* far off.[11] (And the sticks were individually smaller, so the shorter baking time was a function of their size.)

We were befuddled. The cost of our homemade version was less than the convenience product's. The calorie count was better. And the time-for-cooking was certainly in the ballpark. (In fact, as we go through this journey, we can prove this same conclusion again and again with hamburgers, cole slaw, steaks, and chicken breasts.)

So what was stopping everyone from making their own oven-fried fish fillets?

I called our friends with the kids. "What's the deal with those fish sticks?" I asked. "You guys are great cooks. Can't you make your own?"

After I debunked cost and time, they came back with one answer: "Effort."

Effort: a rather hard-to-pin-down variable that expresses how much energy it takes to do something. After months of working on the recipes in this book, of sending them out to our recipe-testers and asking them to conduct similar experiments, Bruce and I have come to one conclusion: when people say they don't have the time to make real food, they really mean they don't want to spend the effort.

Which is sort of crazy, given that it's food we're putting in our bodies. Who doesn't want better fried fish?

OVEN-FRIED FISH FILLETS

Here's Bruce's version from our test case. Try this recipe once and you'll never go back to buying frozen. Just keep this rule in mind when you're buying fresh fish: it should smell fresh, like the ocean on a spring morning at high tide, not like the tidal flats in August.

2 large egg whites

2 tablespoons lemon juice

½ cup yellow cornmeal

½ cup whole wheat flour

1 teaspoon salt

1 teaspoon mild paprika

½ teaspoon dried dill

½ teaspoon freshly ground black
    pepper

1½ tablespoons olive oil

Four 4-ounce skinless, white-fleshed,
    thin fish fillets, such as snapper or
    tilapia

1. Position a rack in the center of the oven and preheat to 400°F.

2. Mix the egg whites and lemon juice with a whisk or a fork in a shallow soup bowl until foamy and well combined.

3. Mix the cornmeal, whole wheat flour, salt, paprika, dill, and pepper in a second shallow soup bowl or on a dinner plate.

4. Drizzle the oil on a large baking sheet, then use a wadded-up paper towel to smear it around.

5. Take one of the fish fillets and dip it in the egg white mixture, coating both sides. Let some of the excess run off, then dip the piece in the cornmeal mixture on both sides. Then do all this again with the same piece of fish: back into the egg white mixture and then back into the cornmeal mixture. Place the fillet on the prepared baking sheet and repeat with the other fillets.

6. Bake for 9 minutes, then use a big spatula to flip the fillets and continue baking for 9 more minutes. Transfer each fillet to a dinner plate and serve while hot.

MAKES 4 SERVINGS

A Plea for Effort

Heaven knows, Bruce and I are often so tired we can barely move by 6:00 p.m. And dinner is an easier thing for us because chances are, Bruce has been cooking all day. We can just pick at the leftovers.

And herein lies the hypocrisy of many a food writer: the hectoring blather of *why don't you just get a nice dinner on the table?* Easily said and done when you cook for a living.

However, that irritating duplicity doesn't mitigate this basic truth: the amount of effort we put into making real food will pay off in better health, better weight maintenance, and better all-around contentment. In a recent shocker, a USDA-backed study showed that people of normal weight spend *more* time shopping for and cooking food than do people who are overweight.[12]

So effort is never to be discounted. That said, there are a few ways to put it in without the task's getting out of hand:

1. Plan ahead.
Make a shopping list; decide what you're going to have for dinner tomorrow night today. We know so many people who say, "But I don't know what I'll want to eat tomorrow." Listen, is this the last meal you'll eat? If not, then it's fine to make a plan and stick to it, even if you find yourself not in the mood for fish on an average Wednesday night. Besides, as you prepare the fish, you'll get in the mood for it, the mere sight of the fresh food instigating hunger the way it should.

2. Avoid the lines.
Explore Fresh Direct, Peapod, and other services that do the shopping for you. No, you won't be able to pick out the cabbage of your choice. But a little compromise is well worth it in the face of crazy schedules.

3. Don't bite off more than you can chew.
Maybe this week you can make only two or three dinners at home. Great! Set that as your goal. Be realistic but also push the boundaries a bit.

And as you're thinking about how you can put in a little more effort for a big result, always focus on real food—as well as the goal of a healthier, thinner, more content you.

A Sense of Accomplishment

Effort makes food an accomplishment, not just a necessity—and that allows for even greater satisfaction. In fact, cooking food ourselves can give rise to the most pleasurable state of effort imaginable: flow.

Long studied by Mihaly Csikszentmihalyi of Claremont Graduate University, flow is a psychological state we all experience from time to time: that moment when the challenge before us and our skills to meet it are wonderfully balanced. Time evaporates; we forget the daily worries; our attention focuses like a beam.

It can happen when we're playing the piano, when we're practicing yoga, or when we're deeply engaged in a conversation. It's the sweet balance of effort and reward.[13]

I watched Bruce become immersed in flow the other day. He was developing a recipe for Mapo Dofu, a Chinese braise of pork, hot chiles, tofu, and tomatoes—a classic dish, but this time a little less heavy. He was trying to figure out the right blend of spices, bending over the bottles in his spice drawer, smelling combinations in the palm of his hand. (You'll find the results of his testing later in this book.)

I came in to ask him a question about the exact deadline for an article and he barely registered my presence. "Soon," he said—as if that meant something.

I didn't press it. He was having the time of his life: creative, in a state of flow.

Cooking itself can be enjoyable, a way to experience life fully and to be creative for a real reward. It can lead to flow.

On the way home from work, anticipate the pleasure of cooking dinner. It's a way to step away from the hassles, do something for yourself, and be creative without anyone looking over your shoulder.

Think about pouring that glass of wine and getting out the onion to chop. Imagine that wonderful sizzle when it hits the oil or butter. Then get home, take the phone off the hook—that means the BlackBerry, too—and start fulfilling that dream.

For more ways to find flow in cooking, try these:

✦ Put on some good music. I'm all Bach; Bruce is Sondheim. To each his own.

✦ Get the lights right. Sounds silly, but we noticed a big difference in how long we stayed in the kitchen when we did no more than put a dimmer switch on the wall for the overhead lights. There's no more glare, now a softer glow.

✦ Get in some comfortable clothes. Neither of us will cook in a tie. Some evils are unspeakable.

✦ Make the space comfortable, too. Who can work on counters loaded with jars, bottles, and other culinary whatnots? Give yourself a nice work surface.

✦ Have someone else around. If I'm not cooking, I'm still in the kitchen with Bruce. I sit on the floor with the dog lying against my legs. We chat, we sing, we rehearse life's foibles. It's what makes a home, every minute of it.

A Clean Slate to Make Dinner

As Bruce and I began to come to terms with the real food chart, we went back into the kitchen, this time to do some housecleaning—or fridge-cleaning, as the case might be. We consulted the chart, read labels, and chucked stuff out. Like these:

✦ Light Mayonnaise (listed ingredients on the bottle: *water, soybean oil, vinegar, modified cornstarch, whole eggs and egg yolks, sugar, salt, xanthan gum, lemon and lime peel fibers, sorbic acid, calcium disodium EDTA [used to protect quality], lemon juice concentrate, phosphoric acid, DL alpha tocopheryl acetate [vitamin E], natural flavors, beta carotene*)

✦ That pear and those celery stalks that had seen better days

✦ That half a candy bar

But we didn't throw out everything. The crackers were Finn Crisp Hi-Fibre Wholegrain Crispbread with Rye Flour. They were a little soggy from being in the refrigerator's chill (I still don't know who put them in there), but we could crisp them up on a baking sheet in a 300°F oven for a few minutes. Plus, we looked at their stated ingredients: *whole-grain rye flour, rye bran, water, yeast, and salt.* Yes, the flour is refined, but it's a whole-grain product and so certainly doesn't fall into the *not real food* category (nor even the *barely real food* category—but that's a story for "Step 6").

Other things we kept included the following:

✦ Marque Guyanese Pride Brand Guyana Hot Crushed Pepper Sauce (listed ingredients on the bottle: *peppers, vinegar, spices, salt*)

✦ Pickapepper Sauce (listed ingredients on the bottle: *tomatoes, onions, sugar, cane vinegar, mangoes, raisins, garlic, salt, peppers, thyme, and cloves*)

✦ Bon Maman Apricot Preserves (listed ingredients on the bottle: *apricots, cane sugar, fruit pectin, citric acid*—pectin is a naturally occurring thickener, what your grandmother would have used to make apricot preserves)

✦ The fat-free milk and the low-fat yogurt (despite appearing "diet-y," neither had anything fake in the mix)

Bruce and I encourage you to do the same. Look through your refrigerator and pantry, then toss out some of the things you don't deem as real food, using the chart in this book and the parameters we've established.

There's no reason to be wasteful. Remember there are two nuanced categories: *almost real food* and *barely real food.* The benefit of the doubt is not the worst thing at this moment. The worst thing is not finding satisfaction in our food—which makes us eat more and more to compensate.

But a step in the right direction is worth a thousand words. So off to the fridge and pantry with you! And once you get it cleaned out, you'll know what you have on hand to help you make a shopping list for a couple of these meals that'll keep it real at the table.

THE PERFECT SALAD

This salad is a meal in every bite: bacon, egg, the works. That poached egg will slowly melt into the dressing, a rich treat guaranteed to slow things down for dinner.

4 cups frisée, stem removed, the leaves roughly chopped (see Notes, page 28)

2 ounces nitrate-free or uncured bacon, chopped

2 medium shallots, minced

2 teaspoons Dijon mustard

1 teaspoon Worcestershire sauce

3 tablespoons white wine vinegar

2 large eggs

Freshly ground black pepper, to taste

1. Place the torn frisée in a large bowl. Meanwhile, bring a large saucepan of water to a simmer.

2. Heat a skillet over medium heat. Add the bacon; cook, stirring occasionally, until frizzled and browned.

3. Stir in the shallots. Cook, stirring often, until softened.

4. Whisk—don't stir—in the mustard and Worcestershire sauce. Then remove the skillet from the heat and whisk in the vinegar. Pour this mixture over the frisée and toss well. Divide the dressed frisée between two plates.

5. Reduce the heat under the water so that it simmers slowly. Crack an egg into a small cup, then gently pour it into the water. Do the same with the second egg on the other side of the saucepan. Turn off the heat and cover the saucepan for 4 minutes.

6. Remove the eggs from the warm water with a slotted spoon, letting the water drain so as not to turn the salad soggy. Set an egg on each salad. Give each a few generous grinds of pepper.

MAKES 2 SERVINGS

(CAN BE DOUBLED FOR A FAMILY MEAL)

ZUCCHINI CAKES

Buy real ricotta: no stretchers, thickeners, or preservatives. It'll make the best patties: fresh, flavorful, and definitely real. Serve these with a little mustard on the side, as well as a light salad, dressed with one of our two new salad dressings (see page 68).

4 medium zucchini

1 teaspoon kosher salt

1 small yellow onion, peeled

½ cup regular or low-fat ricotta

5 tablespoons whole wheat flour

1 large egg, beaten with a fork in a small bowl

½ teaspoon mild paprika

½ teaspoon dried dill

½ teaspoon freshly ground black pepper

1 tablespoon olive oil, plus more as needed

1. Trim the ends off the zucchini, then shred them into a colander, using the large holes of a box grater. (You'll need about 4 cups of shredded zucchini.)

2. Sprinkle the shredded zucchini with salt, toss well, and set it in the sink for 15 minutes to drain.

3. Rinse the zucchini shreds under cool water in the colander. Then pick up in handfuls and squeeze them over the sink to get rid of almost all of the moisture. It'll take some time—but your forearm probably needed a good workout anyway. Squeeze out all the moisture you can, then set the shreds in a large bowl.

4. Grate the onion into the bowl using the large holes of the box grater. (If you want to avoid onion tears, you can grate the onion using the shredding blade in a food processor.)

5. Stir in the ricotta, whole wheat flour, beaten egg, paprika, dill, and pepper, just until the mixture is uniform and there are no streaks of dry flour anywhere.

6. Heat a large skillet over medium heat. Swirl in the oil, then use a ½-cup measuring cup to scoop up the zucchini mixture and plop it into the skillet, scraping out any mixture left in the cup. Flatten the mixture into a thick cake with the bottom of the cup and continue making more.

7. Cook until lightly browned, about 4 minutes, then turn the patties with a large spatula and continue cooking until lightly browned on the other side and a little firm to the touch, about 4 more minutes. If you can't fit all six into your skillet, you'll need a little more oil for the second batch.

MAKES 6 SERVINGS

SHELL-ON SHRIMP WITH GARLIC CREAM SAUCE

We've already talked about eating with all our senses. This recipe will get your hands involved! Eat the shrimp by slurping the sauce off the shells, then peel them before enjoying. Have a lot of napkins handy! Take your time, enjoy every bite, then finish the meal with a bracing, slightly acidic salad of sliced tomatoes, pitted and sliced nectarines, a little minced red onion, and a drizzle of thick, syrupy balsamic vinegar.

1 tablespoon unsalted butter

2 medium shallots, minced

6 medium garlic cloves, minced

1 tablespoon stemmed thyme leaves
or 2 teaspoons dried thyme

½ teaspoon salt

½ teaspoon freshly ground black
pepper

1½ pounds large, shell-on shrimp
(15 per pound), deveined (see Note)

½ cup white wine, dry vermouth, or
canned reduced-sodium chicken
broth

¼ cup heavy cream

1. Melt the butter in a large skillet over low heat.

2. Add the shallots and garlic; cook slowly, stirring often, until the shallots have softened and start to turn golden, about 3 minutes.

3. Stir in the thyme, salt, and pepper; then raise the heat to medium.

4. Add the shrimp. Toss and stir over the heat until they start to turn pink, about 3 minutes.

5. Pour in the wine, vermouth, or broth. Bring to a full simmer, scraping up any browned bits. Simmer until the liquid in the skillet has reduced to about half its original volume.

6. Pour in the cream, stir well, and bring back to a simmer. Cook, stirring often, until the cream has reduced to a thick sauce, less than 1 minute.

Note: Much of the large shrimp (frozen or thawed) sold in super-markets are already deveined. The package will most likely be so labeled; the shells across the arched back will most certainly be split. To devein a shrimp, follow the steps on pages 19–20, but this time you'll need a pair of kitchen shears to cut through the shell and down into the flesh, starting at the thick end and moving toward the feathery tail.

MAKES 4 SERVINGS

STEP

3

Relish What You Eat

WHAT WILL YOU DO?

Develop a basic reckoning of food choices

Commit to slowing down

Prepare meals designed to help you put that
commitment into practice

~~~~~~~~~

WHAT WILL YOU DISCOVER?

The failures of most diets

How much you have been telling yourself *no*

The value of slower sorts of food

Start by Dumping Any Notion of Deprivation

We're surrounded by low-fat crackers, no-fat yogurt, low-carb ketchup, no-carb mayo, deli subs under however-many calories, fast-food healthy choices. Supermarkets and restaurants are minefields of health claims.

Taken together, these products and their claims have made us a nation of dieters. We're all on the lookout for some sort of a fix, assessing what we eat on at least one sliding scale: fats, carbs, sugars, antioxidants, fiber, omega-3s—you name it.

Which means we don't always make great choices. Take, for example, the Miso-Glazed Salmon at one prominent chain restaurant. The cheery menu describes this entrée as *fresh salmon marinated in miso and baked—served with a delicious miso sauce, snow peas, and white rice.*

Seems like a good choice, right? Except the single serving arrives as a whopping hunk of salmon, slathered in wasabi butter. It tops out at 1,673 calories with 39 grams of saturated fat.

I've ordered it. Hell, I've finished it. Frankly, it was delicious. Or at least the first few bites were. After that, I really don't know. The sheer quantity overwhelmed me as I inhaled the soft, sweet bits. And not only it. Before it appeared, I'd already split the chicken quesadillas with Bruce for an appetizer. And since I thought I'd been *good* ordering chicken (not bacon) and salmon (not something *fried*), I gave in to half a piece of Dulce de Leche Caramel Cheesecake. (Yes, I actually took the other half home.)

The best-laid plans . . . In that one meal, I took in 3,446 calories (running up near two days' worth on the USDA scheme) and 80 grams of saturated fat (running up near four days' worth).

I suspect I'm not alone. Most of us go to restaurants and search for so-called light entrées because we're supposed to, or our friends will think better of us if we do, or we're afraid of anything else on the menu. But even seemingly small portions hide big problems. We might choose the tomato basil soup as *light* luncheon fare. Too bad a single bowl at one popular chain has almost 1,100 calories, about half the USDA's recommended daily intake for an adult.

It's Good to Be Full!

Or so hollered one recent advertising campaign for a series of frozen dinners, ready in minutes from the oven or the microwave. The hulking tally for one of these meals—Roasted Carved Turkey (which sounds sort of healthy) with over 1½ pounds of food (which sounds sort of overwhelming)—crests 1,450 calories with 5,410 mg of sodium (more than twice of the USDA's recommended consumption per *day*) and 26 grams of saturated fat.[1]

Gargantuan portions in a snap: that's what we're eating.[2] While we're all dieting in some way, we're also being sold the bill of goods that we can (and should) eat more and more and more. More crackers per serving. More cereal per serving. More food at all times.

In fact, nothing has befuddled Bruce and me like the question of huge portion sizes in restaurants and the economics of it. We can't figure out a business plan in which the point is to offer us more and more for less and less money. Is it just to get us in the door? The portions get larger; the cost goes down. Shouldn't it be the other way around? Shouldn't they be trying to charge us more for less, like the airlines? We'll leave it to the economists to debate, but we both feel there's a whiff of desperation about the whole thing, a rabid attempt to get us in the door this quarter, no matter what it ultimately means to the business bottom line two years down the road.

Anyway, just look at the change in U.S. consumption *per person* over a thirty-year span:

CONSUMPTION OF	PERCENT CHANGE BETWEEN 1970 AND 2003
fats and oils	+63%
grains	+43%
vegetables	+24%
sugars and sweeteners	+19%
dairy products	+5%
calories daily[3]	+23%

One reason for these dramatic increases is that we *have* to eat more or else the agriculture industry might collapse.[4] More and more production means it's all got to go somewhere. Based on today's methods, one acre of U.S. soil can produce 42,000 pounds of strawberries a year. Who wants shortcake?

So there's the marketing strategy: convince us to eat a lot, sell most of it under some sort of vague health claim, and then tell us to eat even more.

No wonder we all diet. We're eating way too much. We can feel it in our bodies; we can see it in our clothes. So when someone comes along with a plan and says to us, "Hey, you should cut down," we agree. And we should. Except what most of the diet gurus are proposing isn't a matter of cutting down. It's just a matter of depriving ourselves—and plays into the dilemmas already rattling around in our heads.

The First Lie of Deprivation: Something Real Is Actually Evil

Cut down the carbs. Cut out the sugar. Cut out the fat. These are some of the answers.

Listen, if we cut out one type of food, no matter what it is, we'll temporarily lose weight. Period.[5]

Mind you, it's not a bad thing to cut way back on sugar for a week, or avoid fatty salad dressings for a while, or dump the after-work cocktail to save a few calories. But following close on the heels of these good intentions comes the first lie that deprivation diets tell: the food we've temporarily cut out must be evil. It's not *how* we eat but *what* we eat.

While driving to a local orchard to pick cherries the other day, Bruce and I happened to catch a prominent, national radio show. The guest was talking about favorite summer foods. Of course, since taste is connected to memory, the call-ins were mostly about favorite *childhood* summer foods. One woman innocently said she never has a summer gathering without making her mom's favorite tuna-macaroni salad.

To which the show's guest responded in utter horror: "Evil, evil carbs."

Millions of Italians must be wrong, but the woman was undaunted. "Can I use whole wheat pasta?"

He audibly shuddered. "It'll taste awful."

"Well," she said resignedly, "you can get used to anything."

Yes, that's what we want: food we have to *get used to.*

The Second Lie of Deprivation:
Substitute This for That

Now watch this next move. You toss out the offending stuff—the carbs, the fat, the sugars, you name it—and then deprivation diets convince you to compensate with tons of grapefruits (the seventies fad). Or watermelon (the eighties fad). Or blueberries (the nineties fad). Or whole grains (the millennial fad). Or omega-3s (the right-now fad). Or whatever the next *it* food will be.

Or much worse: cut out the offending stuff and then replace it with a fake version of itself. Drop the sugars and replace them with artificial sweeteners—some natural, some fully manufactured, some in a no-man's-land in-between.

Or drop the fat and replace it with a chemically modified starch, a long-chain emulsifier, or one of those engineered fats whose only benefit is a bad case of the runs later in the day.

The Third Lie of Deprivation:
Temporary Results Add up
to Permanent Change

Any deprivation diet will work for a while. Of course. Cut out something that's a normal part of your food choices and you *will* lose weight. But that's not a long-term solution. And it's certainly not a *real food* solution.

Just because something worked for a while doesn't mean it will work forever. Witness the Electoral College.

In truth, we're not losing weight despite the plethora of diet sodas and candies. We're not thinner with fat-free everything on our plates. We're not healthier because a million diet gurus are hawking their plans on a million street corners.

Maybe that's why there's been a rather stinky desperation in the new diet schemes popping up on the market lately. They don't cut out one thing; they cut out practically everything.

Thus, the popularity of the new purge diets. One recently popular version was based on some mythology about thin French women. It had us sipping nothing but leek broth for the first weekend . . . then touted its claims to correctness with the inevitable *See, we lost weight.*[6] Of course we lost weight! Quaffing tepid leek water, who wouldn't lose weight? Besides, maybe certain Parisian women are thin, but most suffer from the same eating and weight problems the rest of us do.[7]

Why would anyone buy into a system based on so many lies? Especially when. . . .

Deprivation Diets Fail

Deprivation is not a motivator. It's a blocking mechanism. And once we remove the block, the pent-up desire goes nuts. Or worse yet, quiets to depression.

Who's going to keep drinking leek water? Or not eating chocolate? Or only eating chicken breasts and a plain baked potato? Or cutting out real sweeteners for the fake stuff? Or cutting out this and that all to take some ridiculous supplement? How can anyone stand it?

We can't. Except that failure is then laid at our feet. If we were to outline almost every diet, they would go like this:

1. mandate a dramatic cutback (carbs, fat, you name it),

2. which works temporarily,

3. which proves the diet is trustworthy,

4. except it fails,

5. so we blame ourselves.

Look at that outline. There's a basic pronoun shift: *it* to *we*. We've bought into a bind where if it doesn't work, *we're* at fault.

But a deprivation diet can't work. We run on pleasure, especially when it comes to taste.[8] We are complex beings, made of the dust of this earth and all that grows in it, beings whose innards reward us with endorphins that add up to *ooo, ah*, and *yes*.[9]

And if our goal is to lose weight, we need to stop boiling dinner in a bag, or going on a fat-flush purge, or doing any of the other unspeakable things all those diets require. Instead, we must get back to a place where food is pleasure—even in a world that has so much of it.

Let's be clear: Bruce and I are not talking about triple-dipper ice cream sundaes and cheeseburgers. Rather, we're talking about that simple peach—and what it brings to the dishes prepared with it. We're talking about the delight of food that retains its natural goodness, nutrients, and taste. We're talking about real food, not fussed up or contrived, but straightforward and pleasurable.

Dreydl knows it. He's our collie—and a handful: willful and addicted to chasing chipmunks into the woods. Since we live in a place where we routinely can't get out of the garage because a 500-pound bear is napping on the driveway, it's not the best strategy to have him running like a maniac through the underbrush. So we enrolled him in an obedience class.

Our first night there, we had to sign a contract that said we would never scold our dog, never hit him, never react in anger. Um, okay. Had they met Dreydl?

The only things we were allowed? Praise and food.

We'll let you guess which one worked better.

Actually, it all worked beautifully at first. Within a week, he was more than happy to stay close because he'd learned that there was a boxed dog biscuit in it for him.

Then he quit. He was back to the underbrush on a daily basis.

We asked the trainer what was up.

"The food," she said, a no-nonsense fortysomething. "Would you eat that biscuit?"

Us? Established food writers?

She sensed our hesitation. "So up the stakes," she said with a harrumph.

We did. We fried up some chicken livers, cut them into tiny pieces, and put those in a baggie.

Dreydl passed two levels of obedience, the star of his class.

That dog knew the right answer: the food has to be deeply satisfying for it to register as its own reward. That processed dog biscuit wasn't worth the effort. *You want me to do what for what?*

Still Feeling Deprived Amid Astounding Abundance

Think about the sheer amount of food available in the world. There are convenience stores, vending machines, restaurants, and grocery stores. Even gas stations sell food. After all, there are tons and tons of strawberries that have to be eaten every day! We can't turn around before we find more to eat.

Bruce and I did a quick count the other day. Driving twenty-nine miles down some rural New England roads to our bank in West Hartford, Connecticut, we passed 122 food-selling establishments, from restaurants to grocery stores.

It's not surprising we're all on some sort of deprivation diet. We go about telling ourselves *no* most of the time.

Sometimes consciously, sure. In New York City a few months ago and on our way for Thai food, we watched a young woman in a business suit falter in front of a lovely bakery, one we've visited several times. She did no more than hesitate, a catch in her stride, as she glimpsed the cupcakes—then she instantly struck back into high gear. Lo and behold, she turned in ahead of us at the very Thai restaurant where we were going! She had told herself *no* because lunch was only minutes away. And reasonably so.

But more often, we tell ourselves *no* unconsciously. Food is survival. If we don't eat, we die. So we're wired to be on the lookout for it, scanning the world for opportunities—even when we're not hungry. Over the years, we've been conditioned to know where food is: that restaurant, that grocery store, that food court at the mall. Put simply, these are constant opportunities for what used to be sheer survival.

Let's say we've just had lunch at a restaurant at the mall: a tuna sandwich and a green salad, for example. We walk out to do some more shopping and pass the food court or one of those little cookie stands. We're not hungry; so deep inside, we tell ourselves *no*.

And we should. We're *not* hungry, despite having seen and registered a food source. Animals do this all the time. We've watched our bear picking at the wild berry brambles in the woods beside our house. He goes through a bush or two, eats a mighty lot, and then moves on. He passes other canes loaded with berries, but he doesn't stop to eat more.

However, here's one real difference between us and our bear: I can tell you with utter certainty he will not pass 122 berry brambles in the next two hours. Our wonderful world of overwhelming food abundance has led us to the strange moment when we're having to practice restraint all day every day over and over again, consciously or subconsciously. We're always telling ourselves *no*.

So our land of abundance actually feels like deprivation. And it's a recipe for disaster. We're an oppositional people. Tell us *no*, and we may never stop. Once we hear *don't*, the pleasure of the table is instantly replaced by a set of rules (or prohibitions). Life then morphs into a particularly silly version of *obey or rebel*. We need only think of those no-carb/all-protein fads of the nineties to watch how the faulty logic plays out. As carbs were demonized, we got off them—only to get back on them with shocking abandon.[10]

Watch people at a buffet—a church supper, a family reunion, a community event, a cookout on a cruise. They dive for the food as if they haven't eaten in days—and won't have any obvious opportunities in the future. Sometimes all that *no* just gives way, especially in social settings where eating is celebrated. Sometimes, after telling ourselves *no* long enough, we want a license to say *yes*.

It's high time we removed the games around food and revamped our choices to enjoy every bite—partly so we can indeed turn away from gargantuan proportions without feeling deprived.

To do all that, we're going to celebrate abundance. Not by eating everything and anything we can. Not by heading for the cookie cart right after lunch. But by making sure that what we eat is real food, glorious and full of genuine flavors. And by finding a meal tomorrow and the next day and the next that fits the same bill.

This is the path to our culinary salvation.

Real Meals to Help Us Forget Deprivation Diets

We can't run away from pleasure. Real satisfaction comes from enjoying the world's bounty in reasonable portions. So settle in for a couple of these meals. Taste for complex flavors, celebrate how they connect to memory, find them with all your senses, and chew beyond the first bite.

Your brain is so quick that you have to figure out ways to relish every bite. Like these:

✦ Breathe. Air pulls essential flavors up into the nose, engaging other parts of the mind with the food. When you take a bite, chew a bit and take a slow breath through your nose. You'll start to register so many different tastes.

✦ Occasionally, push some of the partially chewed food onto the roof of your mouth just behind your front teeth. You'll be pushing it closer to your nose, so you'll experience more complex flavors.

✦ Have something to drink. It will increase the complexity of the flavors dramatically. And the liquid will help get those flavors onto your tongue and up in your nose.

CHEESE TOAST WITH PEARS

This is one of our favorite lunches—we've even carried it with us for a quick meal on the road. Search out a crusty, chunky, whole-grain bread to give you the most chew and taste with every bite. Add some roasted or steamed broccoli, carrots, or cauliflower on the side and you've got dinner!

Eight ½-inch slices whole-grain bread

4 teaspoons Dijon mustard

2 medium Bartlett pears, peeled, cored, and very thinly sliced

2½ ounces finely shredded Swiss cheese, Emmentaler, or Gruyère

1½ ounces finely grated hard cheese like aged Gouda (see Note)

1. Position a rack about 5 inches below the broiler and preheat it. Set the bread on a baking sheet and place the tray on the oven rack so that the toast slices are right under the heating element. Toast the bread on both sides until lightly browned and crunchy.

2. Spread each slice of bread with ½ teaspoon mustard. Top each with the pear slices.

3. Mix the two cheeses in a small bowl, then sprinkle 2 tablespoons over each piece of bread and pear.

4. Place the tray back on the oven rack as before and broil until the cheese melts, turns a little brown, and gets bubbly, about 4 minutes. Transfer the sandwiches to a wire rack and cool a few minutes before eating.

Note: No kitchen should be without a proper scale, sold at most cookware stores and online outlets. Its purpose is not to weigh portion sizes. Rather, it's so we can complete a recipe successfully. For example, cheese is always given by weight: 1½ ounces. More, and the dish will turn greasy; less, it may be dry.

MAKES 4 SERVINGS
(CAN BE HALVED FOR TWOSOMES)

WHITE BEAN SALAD WITH GRILLED TUNA

Here's a make-ahead goodie full of flavor without any fake-outs. For dinner, line a plate with lettuce leaves and spoon the salad on top. Make sure you have a piece of a crunchy baguette on the side.

2 tablespoons olive oil, divided

One 6-ounce tuna steak

2 celery stalks, thinly sliced

1¾ cups canned white beans, drained and rinsed

⅓ cup red onion, chopped

2 tablespoons white wine vinegar

1 tablespoon sage leaves, minced

½ teaspoon salt

½ teaspoon freshly grated black pepper

1. Prepare the grill for high-heat cooking or heat a grill pan over medium-high heat. Smear about 1 teaspoon oil over the tuna steak and set on the grill grate directly over the heat or on the grill pan. Continue cooking, turning once, until an instant-read meat thermometer inserted into the center of the tuna registers 140°F, about 6 minutes, maybe 8 (see Note). Transfer to a cutting board and slice into small cubes. Cool for 5 minutes.

2. Place these cubes in a bowl and stir in everything else, including the remaining oil. Serve at once—or cover and refrigerate for lunch the next day.

Note: No kitchen should also be without an instant-read meat thermometer. The only way to tell if a fish steak or any cut of beef, pork, veal, chicken, or turkey is done is to take its internal temperature. The thermometer will give you a reading in seconds, without its having to be left inside the oven. Gently press the probe into the thickest part of the cut and wait a few seconds for the temperature to register. Always wash an instant-read thermometer before a subsequent use.

MAKES 2 SERVINGS

(CAN BE DOUBLED OR TRIPLED)

LEMON CHICKEN CUTLETS

This easy supper will help you realize that fresh flavors don't need a lot of adulteration. Buy the best black olives you can find, preferably the small ones from Nyons or other varietals from Provence.

Four 5-ounce boneless, skinless
   chicken breasts
6 tablespoons unbleached all-purpose
   flour
1 teaspoon salt
1 teaspoon freshly ground black
   pepper
1 tablespoon unsalted butter, divided

2 tablespoons olive oil, divided
3 tablespoons chopped pitted black
   olives
2 teaspoons grated lemon zest
½ cup dry white wine, dry vermouth,
   or reduced-sodium chicken broth
5 tablespoons lemon juice (the juice
   from about 2 medium lemons)

1. Place a chicken breast between two large sheets of plastic wrap on your work surface, then use the bottom of a heavy saucepan (or the flat side of a meat mallet if you have one) to pound the breast to about ¼ inch thick. Or save yourself the trouble and ask your supermarket's butcher to pound the breasts until they're ¼ inch thick.

2. Mix the flour, salt, and pepper together on a large dinner plate.

3. Unless you have a gigantic skillet that can accommodate all the pounded breasts at once, melt ½ tablespoon butter with 1 tablespoon olive oil in a large skillet over medium-high heat.

4. Dredge two breasts in the flour mixture, coating both sides. Knock off any excess flour. Slip them into the skillet and cook until lightly browned and cooked through (you can slice one open to make sure it's white inside), about 4 minutes, turning once. Transfer the breasts to a serving platter or individual plates.

5. Repeat steps 3 and 4 without cleaning the skillet until all the chicken is cooked.

6. Stir the olives and lemon zest into the skillet; cook for about 20 seconds.

7. Pour in the wine, vermouth, or broth, as well as the lemon juice. Raise the heat to high, and bring the mixture to a full, bubbling simmer, scraping the bottom of the skillet occasionally to get any flavorful brown bits up and into the sauce. Cook for about 1 minute, or until slightly reduced. Pour this wet sauce over the breasts.

MAKES 4 SERVINGS

(CAN EASILY BE HALVED FOR TWOSOMES)

Now That You've Dumped Deprivation, Take off Your Coat Before You Pour the Wine

Once, as Bruce and I were jogging through Dulles Airport, trying to make a connection home, he wanted to grab a coffee, a little caffeine to keep him awake. He walked up to a small kiosk and asked for a medium cup.

"Don't you want something to eat?" the chipper woman asked.

"No, thanks. Tired. Just coffee."

"The sandwiches are fresh," she said, doing her best.

He hesitated.

"I just unpacked them."

Fresh? They're not fresh. They haven't been fresh in days. They arrived at the airport on a truck from a processing plant out beyond the exurbs, already sealed in cellophane, stamped with an expiration date, and stacked in cardboard boxes—which got checked in at the airport's central food facility, made it onto trolleys, maybe sat around for a bit, finally got taken to this woman's kiosk, and dumped behind her chair until she was ready to slice open the case and put them out.

Fresh. Not *I made them.* Or *I saw them being made.* Or even

I know where they were made. Fresh, as in *I just unpacked the box.*

That counts as a sales pitch.

Idle Kitchens, More Food

Even as *fresh* became *freshly unpacked*, the national sport of home kitchen renovations has spawned TV shows, magazines, websites, and an industry of remodeling specialists. What's more, many of us have tricked out our appliances: stainless-steel this, copper that. All of which is sort of odd considering how little anyone cooks at home anymore. Watch this:

✦ Around 1934, we devoted almost two and a half hours a day to cooking at home.

✦ By the fifties, when modern appliances had taken root, we were down to one hour a day.

✦ By the midnineties, with the advent of a battalion of frozen meals, we'd shaved it to fifteen minutes.

✦ And today? In 2010, it's projected that the average American will spend eight minutes a day preparing food at home—not per meal, but for all three, snacks included.[11]

To accomplish the Herculean task of cooking our food in eight minutes, we've turned to a lot of processed or packaged foods. Only 58 percent of our meals use at least one raw ingredient.[12] Milk on cereal counts. Which means that 42 percent of foods cooked at home did not include even one raw ingredient.

We've also turned to a lot of heat-it-up, frozen foods: over $32 billion worth in 2010.[13]

But in all actuality, the growth of frozen foods pales in comparison to the growth of prepared and processed foods. Industry statistics are guarded secrets, but we do know that the U.S. *imported* (not counting what we made ourselves) over $31 billion worth in 2007 while the global market has crested $1.3 trillion.[14]

Walk into any supermarket and look at the growth areas: breads and pastries, deli cases, take-home dinners, and rotisserie chickens. Remember that idea that you should shop the supermarket's perimeter to find the freshest, minimally processed, or least packaged stuff? Now you'll mostly find ready-to-go fare in boxes or on warming trays.

So we've revamped our kitchens, bought better cookware, and gotten buried alive in a blizzard of cookbooks and food shows; but we mostly buy processed and packaged stuff. We have pots and pans our ancestors could have only dreamed of but we rely on a stack of take-out menus.

Bruce and I were recently at a dinner party where our hostess told us she has more than a hundred food blogs bookmarked, sites she reads daily. She then proceeded to put out a lovely dinner prepared entirely by a high-end grocery store.

Listen, nobody wants to go back to 1934. Two and a half hours a day spent cooking? That's nuts. Almost as nuts as eight minutes a day.

Cooking Large, Eating Large

When we do cook, we often cook for dinner parties, birthdays, or holidays. Thanksgiving remains the number one day we get in the kitchen. The meals we prepare are hardly the stuff for weekday evenings. We make platters, not dinner.

To make matters worse, the number of servings a published recipe makes has dwindled while the overall amount of food it produces has increased. In *Mastering the Art of French Cooking*, Julia Child claimed a 3-pound chicken served four. Her lobster recipe for six called for three 1½-pound lobsters.[15]

Today, it's hard to find a 3-pound, uncooked bird at the market. Even the fully cooked, rotisseried birds weigh in around 4 pounds. And a 1½-pound lobster is considered a single serving.

All of which is gobbled down in no time flat. On average, we spend about thirty-nine minutes a day eating food at home. Again, eight minutes preparing it, thirty-nine minutes eating it—for all meals and snacks.

When we order in, heat up a meal, or even cook our own dinner, we tend to sit down with it in front of the TV. Chances are, we're finished before the first commercial break. That's seven to eight minutes.

Which means, given our statistics, that we've got at least thirty-one minutes left over for breakfast, lunch, and snacks.

And If We Eat a Lot at Home . . .

In 1955, twenty-five cents of every dollar spent on food in the United States went to restaurants; today that figure is heading north of forty-six cents, with almost unbelievable growth expected in the next decade.

That's not the only thing that's grown. Portion sizes in fast-food restaurants are between two and five times larger than in the mid-1980s.[16]

A recent scholarly article made no bones about it: "Large portions of energy-dense foods can lead to excess energy intakes." In other words, when we're served bigger portions of high-fat, high-sugar foods, we eat more—and gain weight.[17]

I called one of the authors, Barbara J. Rolls, professor of Nutritional Sciences at Penn State and author of the best-selling *Volumetrics Eating Plan*, to follow up. "Most of us have good intentions," she said, "but we have to work hard not to overeat these days. Eventually, if you're serious about taking control of what you eat, you start to find it really hard to go out."[18]

Bruce and I remember growing up in the sixties when portions were not as large as they are now. Take juice, for example. When we were kids, orange juice came in a narrow, squat glass, no more than 2 ounces. It was a treat—expensive and usually freshly squeezed.

Today, it's an expected part of brunch—in an 8-ounce tumbler, if not a 16-ounce one. That small glass when we were kids contained about 28 calories. And the big one today? About 224 calories, probably downed as one beverage among several.

But here's where it really gets surreal. For all the fancy presentations, large portions, and multiple beverages, how long do you think the average American spends eating in a restaurant? Just thirteen minutes.[19]

Watch people sometime. They eat with their heads down, bent over their plates. There's little thought to what they're eating. Just like Bruce and I with our breakfast sandwiches at the airport.

And how in the world can restaurants push out that much food so quickly? We know the answers from our burgers near the mall. The ingredients have been precut, presliced, four-fifths (if not completely) premade, pumped with preservatives, then smeared with a thick coating of fat, sugar, and salt to make the patties palatable—not palatable enough to savor, mind you (thirteen minutes, after all), but just palatable enough that we bolt them down and go about our business, temporarily sated, maybe even stuffed, but certainly not satisfied.

It's best summed up by an episode of that popular sitcom *Designing Women*. Mary Jo was once forced to work at a fast-food restaurant because her ex wasn't making his child-support payments. Julia Sugarbaker and the gang ended up helping her out when the restaurant was overwhelmed with a lunch rush—which led to this priceless exchange with a hapless customer ordering a sandwich:

CUSTOMER: "What kind of fish is it?"

JULIA: "Excuse me?"

CUSTOMER: "The fish sandwich? What kind of fish is it?"

JULIA: "It's sort of compressed."

CUSTOMER: "Is it fresh?"

JULIA: "Well, let me put it this way: you're in a Burger Guy; it's compressed fish, breaded and deep-fried. It costs eighty-nine cents. What do you think?"

CUSTOMER (hesitating): "I don't know."

JULIA (quickly): "Yes, it's fresh."

All is not lost. There are four ways to turn away from the cycles of deprivation with overeating as their inevitable rebound yet still come out a winner every time—and find real food to boot.

First, Decide to Slow Down

Bruce and I have slowed down by making small moments with food events part of a daily ritual—because we've decided that we're the sort of people who relish food.

These days, I eat breakfast every morning. By which I mean that I sit down and eat it. (Isn't it weird that I have to make that qualification?) I love café au lait, a big bowl of espresso with frothed milk. I got tired of hunting for it at coffee shops (it's embarrassing in my PJs), so I bought my own machine. Now, I set my alarm early to have my coffee and read the newspaper. I enjoy a piece of buttered toast (dipped in café au lait, it's sheer ecstasy!) and I'm ready for the day.

Bruce is an on-the-go type: he rolls out of bed and jumps to work. I've seen him go from sleeping to braising in under five minutes. His quiet moments come in the late afternoon. He pours himself a beer, gets a handful of nuts, and heads out to the deck to settle in for some downtime with the birds in the trees.

That's the key: to decide. Imagine yourself as a person who slows down, who takes time with what you eat. Hold that image for a minute. What would that mean for your day? What would that mean for your meals? What would that mean for your spouse, your children, your partner, or your boyfriend?

Second, Learn How to Shape a Meal

Aristotle once wrote that a good story must have a beginning, a middle, and an end. Meals are like that, too: they go from a beginning (we're hungry) to a happy ending (we're satisfied). So here's how to make your meal a memorable story.

When you sit down, do something that indicates you're at the beginning. Some people say a prayer; others say a stock phrase like *bon appétit* or *here's to your health*. Bruce and I often begin with a poem from one of our favorite modern poets: Billy Collins, Philip Levine, or Kay Ryan. We once spent a year reading Shakespeare sonnets before our meals.

The middle? Well, that's what we're all about in this book—learning to enjoy every bite.

Then set an end to your meal, a ritual that tells you dinner is over. Don't just use the TV commercial breaks.

The most common ending is a cup of coffee or tea. But there are other ways you can end meals: a kiss, a hug, a thank-you, a song. Make it a ritual so it has the ring of a conclusion. I know one family who says a prayer after dinner, not before.

As a bonus, giving dinner an end point also helps stop mindless eating afterward. A meal is not an open-ended project.

Third, Choose Foods That Bring on More Satiety

Some foods stave off hunger by manipulating our metabolism and digestive systems so we feel sated for longer. They slow us down internally. You've probably noticed some as repeated ingredients in Bruce's recipes—and you'll see them again in the steps ahead. Here are the top four:

Chiles

They pack a wallop because of a chemical called capsaicin (technically, $C_{18}H_{27}NO_3$), found not in the seeds as people think but instead in little packets in the fleshy veins that run down the inside walls. When cut or even jostled, these packets pop, coating the adjacent seeds with the hot stuff (thus the myth is born). Why this elaborate fandango? Capsaicin is a natural weapon. Birds are immune: they peck at the chiles, digest the seeds whole, and spread them far and wide. We (and all mammals) grind the seeds with our molars and thus stop the plant's propagation—so we're smacked by the chemical defense. Besides the obvious burn on the tongue, one of capsaicin's other biochemical defenses is to trigger signals in our bodies that suppress the appetite, encouraging us to eat less (thus, saving more chiles for the birds).

Ginger
This root has been found to increase the PH of our digestive system, thus decreasing the acidity and helping retard the recurrent flow of gastric juices. As a bonus, there's no pain, as with chiles; ginger is just sweet and delicious. Plus, it can be frozen in unpeeled chunks for up to a year, so you'll always have some on hand.

Pine Nuts
A flavorful addition to so many dishes, these edible seeds from certain pine tree species cause the release of cholecystokinin, a hormone that yields gut-level feelings of satiety and contentment. In other words, you feel fuller and want to eat less.

Broccoli
Your mother was right: eat your broccoli. And not only broccoli but all leafy greens. They aid digestion and offer complex gastric reactions that lead you to satiety faster. Sure, a steak might make your brain happy, but broccoli actually makes your stomach happier. And learning to get in touch with what's going on down there, learning to let those neurons do some of the talking, is a sure step toward better health—and greater contentment.

Mentioning these four ingredients brings up an important point about what we eat in general: not all calories are created equal. Convincing ourselves to slow down is a worthy goal for increasing satisfaction. But if the food we eat leaves us still hungry or unfulfilled, all our good intentions are for naught.

Remember when Bruce and I wolfed down those burgers at the chain restaurant and were eyeing the muffins a few hours later? To figure out what was going on, let's imagine you and I actually sat down to eat two different meals, each with the same number of calories. Which would hold us the longest before hunger struck again?

+ a 5-ounce chicken breast, sautéed in a small skillet with 1 tablespoon olive oil, as well as a medium-baked potato and a medium apple—and go ahead, use a couple tablespoons of chutney with the chicken, put a tablespoon of butter on the baked potato, drizzle the apple slices with a couple teaspoons of honey, and give everything a little salt and freshly ground black pepper

+ a medium bag of gumdrops (about 6½ ounces)

Unfair, you might say.

Is it? Remember: both meals have about the same number of calories.[20] Which are just units of energy. Every one is equal to every other by the laws of physics. So both meals should hold us the same amount of time. Yet we know the first meal will last us several hours, whereas the gumdrops will leave us hungry in no time flat, even if we take half an hour and chew every piece forty times.

The difference is caused by the way food is digested, by the way it leaves our stomachs. Calories may be equal in science but they're not in our bellies. Protein and fiber leave our stomachs slowly— protein, for example, at a rate of about 4 calories per minute.[21] Which means that our chicken breast meal, packed with natural fiber in the baked potato and the apple, even with the added fat and sugar (the butter and the honey), is going to hold us longer than the same number of calories from a bag of gumdrops.

So we don't just need to slow down; we must also choose foods that will stick with us for longer periods of time. And here's part of the answer: protein and fiber.[22] A sandwich that's mostly a big hit of sugars (in the form of refined carbs in the bread and corn syrup in the spreads) isn't going to hold us for very long at all.[23]

Here's another comparison:

+ 2 cups cooked brown rice, a tablespoon of butter, some salt and pepper

✦ One 4-ounce, king-size candy bar

Again, the calories are about the same.[24] Yet we know, despite their ads to the contrary, that candy bars simply won't hold us. That's because sugar empties out of our stomachs at a very fast rate, at about 10 calories per minute—whereas the high fiber in the brown rice will hold us a while.

Let's be clear: Bruce and I are not saying anyone needs to go eat a plate of brown rice for lunch. Ick! But we need to start thinking about ways to hold off hunger and increase satisfaction. Fiber sticks around and keeps us content.

We should always up the fiber in what we eat. Ask for the sprouts with the sandwich; choose the whole-grain bread. Ask for some crunchy carrots or celery on the side. Eat an apple or half a whole wheat muffin for a snack. Add more beans or chickpeas to a salad rather than cheese and sweet dressings. A lunch of soft pasta and cheese sauce will not hold us until dinner.

Now it's going to get outrageous. Here's a final comparison:

✦ that 4-ounce, king-size candy bar

✦ half a 7-ounce bag of potato chips

Ah, this one's tougher. But we probably know the answer just from feeling it in our bellies. The potato chips will actually hold us longer, despite their having about 10 percent fewer calories than the candy bar. That's because fat empties out of the stomach at a rate similarly slow to protein and fiber.[25]

Which can be a problem. We can eat a lot of fat and feel very satisfied, held back from hunger for hours. In fact, restaurants often pump up the fat to increase their customers' satiety. But fat is terribly high in calories; a good way to put on excess pounds in no time.

We'll get to a fuller answer to this dilemma in the steps ahead. For now, let's just say that we want to think about increasing fiber (think vegetables and whole grains), having some good protein, and even adding a little fat to our meals—all to increase satisfaction and keep hunger at bay. Like one of these two meals:

LENTIL, PEAR, AND WALNUT SALAD

Here's a stick-with-you meal, especially alongside crunchy radishes and a sliced cucumber. There's natural fat in the walnuts, as well as lots of fiber in the lentils—and even in the sweet pear. Lentils are done quickly, so take care not to overcook them. If you don't want to buy a bag of carrots or a whole head of celery, look for individual carrot stalks and celery ribs at the salad bar of your supermarket.

1½ cups dry brown lentils, rinsed and picked over for stones

1 ripe pear, halved, cored, and finely chopped

1 medium carrot, peeled and finely chopped

1 medium celery rib, finely chopped

½ cup walnut pieces, finely chopped

¼ cup walnut oil

3 tablespoons cider vinegar

2 teaspoons stemmed thyme

½ teaspoon salt

½ teaspoon freshly ground black pepper

1. Put the lentils in a large pot, add water until it's about 2 inches over the top of them, and bring to a boil over medium-high heat, stirring occasionally. Reduce the heat to low, and simmer until the lentils are tender but with still a little resistance when bitten, stirring occasionally, about 10 minutes. Drain in a colander set in the sink.

2. Pour the lentils into a large serving bowl; stir in everything else.

MAKES 4 SERVINGS

SKILLET MACARONI AND BROCCOLI AND MUSHROOMS AND CHEESE

By increasing the fiber in this casserole (both with whole wheat pasta and more veggies), we can enjoy the luxury of a down-home favorite. This isn't a baked casserole but a skillet supper, quicker and easier.

6 ounces grated Cheddar cheese

2 ounces finely grated Parmigiano-Reggiano

1 tablespoon unsalted butter

1 small yellow onion, chopped

6 ounces cremini or white button mushrooms, sliced

3 tablespoons unbleached all-purpose flour

3 cups low-fat or fat-free milk

1 tablespoon Dijon mustard

1 tablespoon minced tarragon leaves or 2 teaspoons dried tarragon

½ teaspoon salt

½ teaspoon freshly ground black pepper

8 ounces dried, whole wheat pasta shells (not the large ones for stuffing), cooked and drained according to the package instructions

4 cups broccoli florets and stems (see Note)

1. Mix the Cheddar and Parmigiano-Reggiano in a medium bowl. Set aside.

2. Melt the butter in a large, high-sided, oven-safe skillet. Add the onion and cook, stirring often, until softened, about 3 minutes.

3. Add the mushrooms and cook until they release their liquid, it comes to a simmer, and then reduces by about two-thirds, about 5 minutes.

4. Sprinkle the flour over the vegetables in the skillet. Stir well to coat.

5. Whisk in the milk in a steady, thin stream until creamy. Then whisk in the mustard, tarragon, salt, and pepper. Continue whisking until the mixture starts to bubble and the liquid thickens, about 3 minutes.

6. Remove the skillet from the heat. Stir in three-quarters of the mixed cheeses until smooth. Then stir in the cooked pasta and the broccoli.

7. Preheat the broiler after setting the rack 4 to 6 inches from the heat source. Meanwhile, sprinkle the remaining cheese over the ingredients in the skillet. Set the skillet on the rack and broil until

light browned and bubbling, about 5 minutes. (If your skillet has a plastic or wooden handle, make sure it sticks outside the oven, out from under the broiler, so the handle doesn't melt.) Cool for 5 to 10 minutes before dishing up.

Note: Broccoli florets can be cut off the larger stalks. (Save the chopped stalks in the freezer to be used for stews.) Make sure the florets are small: an inch across at the largest. If larger, drop them into the pasta water to cook for 1 minute. Drain in a colander set in the sink with the pasta and just dump both into the skillet in step 6.

MAKES 4 SERVINGS

~~~~~~~

Finally, Grow with the Flow

We've already talked about finding a sense of accomplishment in the kitchen, of treating it as a pleasurable act of creation in the state of flow. But we can only maintain flow if we keep pushing the boundaries.

Boredom can be standard operating procedure when we cook. Most evenings, we're dead tired and set the challenge far too low, resorting to the same old recipes or foods. Not only are we uninterested, the food we cook is uninteresting. Our palates suffer, caught in tedium. There's no flow anywhere in sight, nor even the possibility of it.

To compensate, we sometimes shoot too high. We dive headfirst into a whole complicated mélange, buying flaxseeds and quinoa and things we've never heard of, roasting this and braising that, a sort of frenzy to be on top of the game.

Soon enough, frustration sets in. It's too hard, too far, too much. Caul fat what? Mince how? Every turn reminds us of how far we have to go—although we're pretending to be at the end of the course already. So we throw in the towel, glad to be done.

Flow can be achieved only when our skills and their challenges are growing over time. As Csikszentmihalyi writes, flow's end result, its whole point (as it were), is "growth and discovery."[26] This means we must always be expanding the challenge. Otherwise, we'll find ourselves bored and back on the processed, packaged merry-go-round.

So Bruce and I want to start increasing your skills in the kitchen, pushing you a bit so you'll find more enjoyment in preparing your meals. To that end, here are four recipes, each based on a classic cooking technique. You can hone your skills and maybe learn a thing or two, always the key to greater enjoyment at what you do.

SAUTÉED CHICKEN BREASTS PUTTANESCA-STYLE

From the French word for "to jump," sautéing involves browning meat, fowl, fish, or shellfish in a hot skillet. The food skitters and sizzles, sort of jumping as it browns. Which is really the point. Give these chicken breasts enough time over the heat to get a uniform, browned look. That caramelized flavor will permeate the meat—and lie in little burned bits on the skillet's bottom, waiting to be lifted off with this classic sauce of tomatoes, olives, and capers.

Four 5-ounce boneless, skinless chicken breasts	3 medium garlic cloves, minced
½ teaspoon salt	½ teaspoon red pepper flakes
½ teaspoon freshly ground black pepper	¼ cup sliced pitted black olives
1 tablespoon olive oil	1 tablespoon capers, drained, rinsed, and chopped
1 tablespoon unsalted butter	1¾ cups canned reduced-sodium diced tomatoes (one 15-ounce can)

1. Heat a large nonstick skillet over medium heat. Meanwhile, season the chicken breasts with salt and pepper.

2. Swirl the olive oil into the skillet, then slip the chicken breasts in and cook until well browned, about 6 minutes. Don't skimp—

you want lots of color for lots of flavor. The breasts may well stick at first but let them keep browning and searing over the heat. Soon enough, you'll be able to pop them up with a large spatula, the natural sugars and proteins releasing from the hot surface.

3. Turn the breasts and continue cooking until well browned on the other side, about 5 more minutes, until an instant-read meat thermometer inserted into the center of one breast registers 165°F. Transfer to a plate.

4. Melt the butter in the skillet, then add the garlic and red pepper flakes. Stir over the heat until aromatic, about 20 seconds.

5. Add the olives and capers, then pour in the tomatoes. Bring to a simmer, scraping up any browned bits on the skillet's bottom. Knock the heat down to low and simmer slowly until the sauce has thickened a little, about 3 minutes. Basically, if you run a wooden spoon through the sauce, it'll hold that line a second or so before flowing back into place.

6. Return the breasts and any accumulated juices on their plate to the skillet. Cook for about 2 minutes, just until the breasts are warmed through.

MAKES 4 SERVINGS

FISH FILLETS IN PACKETS

Despite the use of fussy parchment paper, found near the aluminum foil and wax paper at the supermarket, no technique is easier than this classic method that seals food in packets and then bakes it in a hot oven, creating a little steam chamber, no extra fat needed. Although this recipe makes a single serving, you can make as many packets as you need for as many as you have to feed by multiplying the ingredients at will. Lift the packets right off the baking sheet with a large spatula, then set each one on a plate, letting everyone peel open their own. Careful of that hot steam!

One 16-inch aluminum foil sheet

One 16-inch parchment paper sheet

1 tablespoon oregano leaves, minced

One 5- to 6-ounce skinless, thin-fleshed fish fillet such as haddock, snapper, bass, or red trout

½ cup yellow summer squash or zucchini, diced

3 cherry tomatoes, quartered

2 jarred artichoke hearts packed in water, drained and quartered

1 tablespoon dry white wine, dry vermouth, or 2 teaspoons water plus 1 teaspoon lemon juice

½ teaspoon salt

½ teaspoon freshly ground black pepper

1. Position a rack in the center of the oven and preheat to 450°F.

2. Lay the sheet of aluminum foil on your work surface, then top with the sheet of parchment paper. Sprinkle the oregano in the center of the sheet, then set the fillet on top.

3. Sprinkle the yellow squash or zucchini, cherry tomatoes, artichoke hearts, wine or its substitute, salt, and pepper over the fillet.

4. Fold and crimp the packet closed, making sure there are no gaps anywhere. The best way is to crimp the two long edges closed by folding them over each other a couple times, then pinching them tightly shut. Roll up the short edges, taking care not to reopen the long, central seam.

5. Place the packet on a large baking sheet; bake for 15 minutes. Let stand at room temperature on the baking sheet for 5 minutes before serving.

MAKES 1 SERVING

BRAISED LAMB SHANKS WITH LEMON AND WHITE BEANS

A braise involves long-stewing tough cuts of meat and root vegetables in a little liquid, less than you would for a stew. In effect, there are two techniques at once: simmering the parts submerged in the liquid and steaming those resting above, the better to allow the meat's natural collagen and fat to melt into an incredible sauce. It isn't much work, other than to wait for the dish to get done.

1 tablespoon olive oil

6 lamb shanks (about 4½ pounds in all)

1 large yellow onion, chopped

3 medium carrots, chopped

1 cup white wine, dry vermouth, or
   ½ cup unsweetened apple juice
   mixed with ½ cup reduced-sodium
   chicken broth

2 tablespoons finely grated lemon zest

2 tablespoons minced sage leaves or
   1 tablespoon dried sage

1½ teaspoons salt

1 teaspoon celery seeds

½ teaspoon freshly ground black
   pepper

2½ cups white beans, drained and
   rinsed, divided

1½ cups reduced-sodium fat-free
   chicken broth

¼ cup lemon juice

1. Heat a large Dutch oven over medium heat. Swirl in the oil, then add the shanks (in batches, if necessary, to avoid crowding) and brown all over, about 8 minutes in all. Transfer to a plate.

2. Add the onion and carrot; cook, stirring often, until the onion has begun to turn translucent and smells sweet, about 4 minutes.

3. Stir in the wine or its substitute, lemon zest, sage, salt, celery seeds, and pepper; raise the heat to high and bring to a full simmer. Cook until the liquid has reduced to about half its original volume.

4. Stir in 1½ cups of the beans, as well as the broth; return the shanks and any accumulated juices to the pot.

5. Bring to a full simmer; then cover, reduce the heat to low, and simmer slowly until the lamb is tender when poked with a fork at its large "knuckle" end, about 2½ to 3 hours.

6. Use a fork to mash the remaining 1 cup of beans and the lemon juice into a paste in a small bowl. Stir the mixture into the simmering sauce and cook for 1 minute, just to warm through.

MAKES 6 SERVINGS

STIR-FRIED GENERAL TSAO'S VEGETABLES

Stir-frying is all about cooking ingredients quickly without too much caramelization. Thus, it always involves (1) prepping everything in advance so you can work like mad over the heat, and (2) using Asian condiments to make a flavorful sauce without any browning—in the case of this dish, bottled oyster sauce, soy sauce, and rice vinegar, all available in the Asian aisle of your market. Serve the dish over cooked brown rice or steamed baby bok choy (chopped into chunks and washed to remove any sand).

1 tablespoon sesame oil

4 medium scallions, thinly sliced

1 tablespoon peeled minced fresh ginger or jarred preminced ginger

2 medium garlic cloves, minced

1 teaspoon red pepper flakes, or to taste

1 pound shiitake mushroom caps, thinly sliced (do not use the stems—they are too fibrous)

1 pound green beans, chopped

2 medium yellow squash or green zucchini, roughly chopped

2 medium carrots, shredded through the large holes of a box grater

2 tablespoons oyster sauce

2 tablespoons reduced-sodium soy sauce

2 tablespoons rice vinegar (see Note)

1 teaspoon packed light brown sugar

1 teaspoon cornstarch stirred with 1 tablespoon water in a small bowl, optional

1. Heat a large, nonstick wok or sauté pan over medium-high heat for 2 minutes.

2. Swirl in the oil, then add the scallions, ginger, garlic, and red pepper flakes. Stir and toss over the heat for 20 seconds.

3. Add the mushrooms, green beans, squash, and carrots. Stir and toss over the heat until the vegetables have begun to get tender but still have a little crunch, about 3 minutes.

4. Pour in the oyster sauce, soy sauce, vinegar, and sugar. Stir well until bubbling, about 30 seconds. If you like a thicker sauce, add the cornstarch mixture and toss over the heat just until the sauce thickens, about 20 more seconds.

Note: An Asian staple, rice vinegar is made from rice wine. It comes in two varieties: unseasoned and seasoned. Seasoned has sugar in the mix—and is often labeled *seasoned*, even in tiny type. The more standard, unseasoned bottling is not so marked. But sometimes, the only way to tell is to read the ingredient list. The recipes in this book call for only the standard, unseasoned variety.

MAKES 4 SERVINGS

4

Detox Your Palate from Useless Salt, Fat, and Sugars

WHAT WILL YOU DO?

Prepare some meals without salt at all—
and some enhanced by better salt
Learn how to get more satisfaction from fats
Enjoy sweet accents in food without guilt or fear
Make a great burger

~~~~~~~~~

WHAT WILL YOU DISCOVER?

The effects of sodium
Better types of salt
Why we need fat
The biological drive for sweet
The two real sweeteners

A Trojan Horse

In the food we enjoy, there's:

✦ what we eat

✦ and what we use to enhance what we eat

What we eat? That's easy enough. Take a package of boneless, skinless chicken breasts. They'll be the centerpiece of our main course. "We're having chicken breasts for dinner."

But we're not. Or not exclusively. We've singled out the basic ingredient *(what we eat)* and overlooked the things that can make it more pleasurable:

✦ salt to make the flavors more distinct

✦ fat to instigate both good cooking and the necessary cues to satisfaction

✦ condiments, mostly sweet, to add depth and sophistication

Those enhancements are all well and good—except they can also become the little soldiers lurking inside the Trojan Horse that is our dinner.

We don't even know they're in there—*We're having chicken breasts for dinner*—but they can quickly take over. Food becomes little more than a vehicle for salt, fat, and added flavors.

Should we go back to plain ol' chicken breasts? Of course not. We love salty, rich, sweet flavors.

But there's a lot of research to suggest that we overeat because we mistake the enhancements for the food itself.[1] So in this step, we're going to take these enhancements one by one, trying to figure out how we can return them to their proper place and thereby find more pleasure in what we eat.

The First Detox: Salt

We crave salt because we need it.[2] Nature's funny that way.

But not all of it. Salt is sodium chloride, a sodium atom and a chlorine atom in one molecule. We crave the sodium part—which balances our bodies' fluids, aids in nerve transmissions, and affects muscular contraction.

We leak sodium when we're sick, particularly during digestive distress. Therefore, many doctors recommend salty drinks like Gatorade. The sodium attracts water to the blood, water that then goes straight to our muscles and organs, rehydrating them when they're under stress.

Salt is just as powerful on our dinner plates. It suppresses bitter and unwanted notes, thereby giving our taste buds easier access to the flavors we prefer.[3]

It also allows us to accomplish culinary techniques that might leave our food unpalatable. When we sear meat and vegetables over high heat, we caramelize (that is, break apart) external sugars and proteins.

We savor these shorter, simpler sugars and smaller, snapped-apart proteins more easily than long-chain ones, so we've long learned to identify browning (like grill marks) with flavor.

But there's a problem. Searing actually dries out food. Salt to the rescue! It takes only a pinch to trick us into thinking our steak or chicken is as juicy as it is tasty. We salivate and mistake desiccation for lusciousness.

Neat compensation, eh?

Oven-fried potato chips are a perfect way to watch all that happen.

OVEN-FRIED POTATO CHIPS

The oven's high heat removes a great deal of the chips' moisture. Even so, they're darn tasty, mostly because of the salt.

2 medium-size russet, baking, or yellow-fleshed potatoes (about two ½-pound potatoes—no need to peel)

1 tablespoon olive oil

½ teaspoon kosher salt or sea salt

1. Position a rack in the center of the oven and preheat to 450°F.

2. Slice the potatoes using the 2-mm slicing blade of the food processor. Stand the potato on its narrow end inside the feed chute (so that you'll get more round slices, rather than long, thin ones); push it down and onto the spinning blades. Repeat with the second potato. Alternatively, slice the potatoes on a mandolin using the 2-mm slicing position, creating thin rounds rather than long slices. Or if you have a very sharp knife, you can make very thin rounds from the potatoes (about ten rounds per inch). Make sure they're all exactly the same width or some will burn before the others are finished cooking.

3. Lay paper towels on your work surface, lay the potatoes out in one layer on the paper towels, cover with more paper towels, and press to blot dry.

4. Brush half the oil on the baking sheet—or dab half the oil on a wadded-up paper towel and spread it generously but smoothly over the baking sheet. Uncover the potato slices, place them in one layer on the baking sheet, and brush the slices with the remaining oil (or dab them with the oiled paper towel you used on the baking sheet).

5. Bake for 20 minutes, until lightly browned. Sprinkle the slices with the salt while they're still hot and immediately transfer to a wire baking rack to cool.

MAKES 4 SERVINGS

GETTING MORE THAN OUR FILL OF SALT

Sodium occurs naturally in what we eat—but in smaller quantities than we require. Yes, broccoli has a smidgen in every cell; but we'd need to eat a daily wheelbarrow's worth to get enough. So we seek out an efficient delivery system as a supplement. Table salt fits the bill.

How much should we take in? The National Academy of Sciences, Institute of Medicine estimates we need between 1,500 and 2,400 milligrams (mg) a day. The USDA opts for 2,300 mg a day for most people, with a lower limit of 1,500 mg for the infirm, the aged, African Americans, and those with blood pressure problems. In either case, consider it between ½ and 1 teaspoon a day.

Well, I certainly don't eat a teaspoon of salt every day, you might say. *I never pick up the shaker at the table; I never add more than a recipe requires.*

Maybe not. But the average American downs between 3,500 mg and 4,000 mg each day.[4]

Why's that so bad? Precisely because sodium collects water—which can bloat just about everything: ankles, wrists, and waists for sure, but most pressingly the blood, increasing its volume. Our hearts then have to work harder to pump the excess, leading to high blood pressure and an armada of nasty health problems.

We've got three sources for all that sodium.[5] Here they are in ascending order:

1. 11 Percent from the Shaker

This is the stuff we add at the stove or the table. But even if we took the high end of our sodium consumption (that is, 4,000 mg a day), we'd end up with only 440 mg based on our sprinkling. That's well under any recommended limits.

Still, this is an easy place to practice a little restraint. Here are three tips:

✦ Move the shaker off the table and into the cabinet, letting salt be a culinary enhancement at the stove.

✦ Consider cutting the amount of salt in half for most standard recipes, particularly if they also call for high-sodium products like bacon, ham, or pepperoni.

✦ Taste before you salt. If you want more salt, sprinkle some into your palm, pinch up a few grains, and put it on what you're eating. You'll actually *see* how much you're getting. If you're considerably thirsty thirty minutes after a meal, you've probably had too much sodium. Now you know for the next time.

2. 12 Percent from Food Sources

As we've already indicated, almost all living things store sodium in their tissues. Here's the content of some common foods:

✦ 1 cup sour cherries: 5 mg

✦ ½ cup boiled beets: 40 mg

✦ ½ cup raw sliced celery: 50 mg

✦ 1 large egg: 63 mg

✦ ½ cup steamed spinach: 65 mg

✦ One 4-ounce boneless, skinless chicken breast: 77 mg

✦ 3 ounces steamed shrimp: between 126 and 195 mg, depending on the type

None will break the bank. In fact, if we again argue from the upper limit of American consumption (that is, 4,000 mg a day), we discover we get around 920 mg a day (or 23 percent) from both the shaker and natural sources. We're still doing very well, with some to spare.

So where does the majority of our sodium come from?

3. 77 Percent from Either Prepared or Processed/Packaged Foods

Let's look at them separately.

Prepared Foods

There are few places where salt is added as freely as at restaurants and the prepared food counters of most supermarkets. Not only does it bring out natural sweetness and flavors, it also stabilizes food as it sits in the kitchen.

Almost no restaurant makes what we order when we order it. They assemble. Even four-star establishments prepare sauces and side dishes earlier in the day. But as food sits around waiting for the dinner rush, its taste dulls because of evaporation and the natural breakdown of relatively unstable flavor compounds. The solution? More salt.

Let's go back to those burgers Bruce and I ate at the adult casual restaurant near the mall. I complained that they were very salty. How salty? Well, a quick check of the sodium content for cheeseburgers at top chain restaurants reveals that these sandwiches can pack in between 1,220 mg and 2,190 mg per serving!

You might argue that the cheese is skewing our numbers. True, cheese has sodium, but not as much as you might think. A Kraft American Single has about 320 mg per slice. So cheese is hardly the whole story. Mostly, the patties and buns are contributing to those numbers.

Which are ridiculously high, some ranging near 100 percent of the suggested daily intake—and that's in just one basic cheeseburger, no salty fries, no sodium-laced ketchup, nothing else. And it's only one example among legion. Try the chicken wraps, fish tacos, fried onion flowers, or fettuccini al fredo from some chain restaurants. All contain nearly 2,000 mg per serving.

Always ask a restaurant chef to go light on the salt. You can add more at the table—and thus be in control of your own food.

Processed/Packaged Foods

These include canned foods of all sorts (soup, for example), almost any condiment you can name (ketchup, barbecue sauce, mustard, pickle relish, Worcestershire sauce, hot sauce, salsa, etc.), any boxed cookie, snack, or treat, as well as crackers, cereals of all sorts, and even bottled drinks. A 12-ounce can of carbonated soda has around 40 mg of sodium.

Why so much sodium? Yes, there's our drive for it. But salt is also a preservative. Bacterial problems in food occur largely because of water. Bacteria—like the rest of us—need it to survive. Salt attracts water. Put crudely, it dries out food. So salt and the other sodium derivatives are pumped into what we eat to minimize spoilage.

Sodium is also the base of many chemical thickeners, emulsifiers, and stabilizers used to create processed foods. If you go back and look at the additives we discussed in Step 2, you'll be surprised how many contain sodium.

True, these are unintentional sources of sodium—not added for the taste but as part of some other chemical compound. But regardless of why it's there, we still break it down and ingest it as sodium.

Here are some other common sources of sodium in packaged or processed foods:

SODIUM SOURCE	HOW IT'S MADE	HOW IT WORKS	HOW IT'S USED	REAL FOOD CATEGORY
Baking soda (a.k.a. sodium bicarbonate)	Naturally found in mineral spring deposits but now mostly mined from the Green River Formation in Colorado and Wyoming	Interacts with acids (vinegar, lemon juice, buttermilk, etc.) to form carbon dioxide and create tiny bubbles in batters	Added to baked goods to make them rise. At home you might use no more than ½ teaspoon in a batter: manufacturers often add lots more to ensure that the baked goods rise and stay fresh	Almost real food (in appropriate amounts)

SODIUM SOURCE	HOW IT'S MADE	HOW IT WORKS	HOW IT'S USED	REAL FOOD CATEGORY
Baking powder	A manufactured mix of baking soda (see page 122), an acid salt of some kind (like sodium aluminum sulphate or disodium pyrophosphate), and cornstarch (to prevent clumping)	Because the acid is already in the mix, it only needs a liquid (water, milk) to activate the bubbles	Causes baked goods to rise. It's a cooking tool to be used wisely; again, manufacturers often add more than home cooks (and it's a double hit—sodium bicarbonate *plus* another salt)	Barely real food. (Search out brands without aluminum. Do you *really* need to consume this metal?)
Monosodium glutamate (a.k.a. MSG)	Originally extracted from wheat gluten but now made by fermenting a starch of some kind	Increases the meaty, savory, salty flavors through glutamic acid, a nonessential amino acid	Found in barbecue sauces, salad dressings, seasoning mixes, and many packaged foods (like canned beef broth—see page 41)	Not real food (a fake-out)
Sodium alginate	A gumlike resin extracted from brown algae	Adheres and gells	Used as an emulsifier and even a glue (for example, to secure the pimiento in stuffed olives); also used in many canned foods to maintain a chunky appearance (like in pie fillings, ham salad, or pet food)	Not real food (a fake-out)

SODIUM SOURCE	HOW IT'S MADE	HOW IT WORKS	HOW IT'S USED	REAL FOOD CATEGORY
Disodium phosphate (a.k.a. disodium hydrogen orthophosphate, sodium hydrogen phosphate, or sodium phosphate dibasic)	Chemically manufactured, a sodium salt made from phosphoric acid	Attracts water molecules	Added to packaged batter mixes to keep them powdery—thus, an anti-caking agent. Also a cleaning agent to scrape off hard water deposits	Not real food (a fake-out)
Sodium nitrate or nitrite	Naturally occurring compounds, once found in rocks (thus the original name of sodium nitrate—saltpeter [*petros* being Greek for "rock"])	Added to cured meats to maintain their color and inhibit the growth of botulism	Eventually forms nitric oxide myoglobin, which colors cured or smoked meats pink	A tough call. We list them as *not real food*; others might list them as *barely real food*

If possible, seek out low-sodium alternatives in convenience products. Once again, be in control of your own shaker.

4. Cooking Without Salt

Let's start rethinking our relationship to this real food enhancement by making a few recipes without any salt at all. Why? Because when the other ingredients are already salty, there's no need to add any extra. What's more, when salt is used sparingly, we can taste food more fully: more dominant flavors and subtle overtones shine through.

CHOWDER-STYLE MUSSELS

Briny mussels (or clams or oysters) are high in sodium. You don't need to add any salt to the pot.

1 tablespoon unsalted butter

1 large yellow onion, chopped

2 celery ribs, thinly sliced

1 medium yellow potato, such as a Yukon Gold, diced into very small bits

1¾ cups reduced-sodium vegetable broth

3 tablespoons heavy or whipping cream

1 tablespoon stemmed thyme leaves

4 pounds cleaned and debearded mussels (see Note)

1. Melt the butter in a large pot over medium heat. Add the onion, celery, and potato. Cook, stirring often, until the onion starts to soften a bit, about 3 minutes.

2. Stir in the broth, cream, and thyme. Bring to a full simmer; then cover, reduce the heat to low, and simmer until the little potato cubes are tender, about 10 minutes.

3. Turn the heat to medium-high and stir in the mussels. Bring to a full simmer; then cover, reduce the heat back to low, and simmer until the mussels open, about 5 minutes.

Note: Mussels should smell fresh and briny, never fishy. Some of the shells may be opened but they should close when tapped. At home, store them for no more than 12 hours in your refrigerator in a large bowl loosely covered with damp paper towels. When you're ready to use them, rinse them in cool water, scrubbing the shells lightly with a potato brush or your fingernails to get rid of any sand. Discard any mussels that are open and will not close when gently squeezed. Then debeard them—that is, remove the wiry hairs that sometimes protrude from the shells; pull these off just before you cook the mussels. Once the mussels are cooked, always err on the side of safety and discard any that are not open.

MAKES 4 SERVINGS

Condiments add plenty of sodium—as here, with the Dijon mustard (to go along with the natural sodium in the seafood). What's the secret to keeping salmon burgers moist every time? A little ground shrimp as the binding agent.

2 pounds skinless salmon fillet	2 tablespoons Dijon mustard
¼ pound medium shrimp, peeled and deveined (see Note, pages 19–20)	½ teaspoon freshly ground black pepper
2 to 3 tablespoons stemmed thyme or minced tarragon leaves	2 tablespoons olive oil

1. Cut the salmon into chunks and add them to a large food processor with the shrimp. Pulse a few times, then process just until coarsely ground with some chunky graininess. If you don't have a food processor, you can repeatedly chop the ingredients on a chopping board, gathering the parts of the fish together and chopping the ingredients until the mixture is about the texture of ground beef.

2. Scoop the mixture into a large bowl (be careful of the sharp blade if using a food processor); stir in the thyme or the tarragon, mustard, and pepper. Form into 6 round patties.

3. Heat a large skillet or grill pan over medium heat. Swirl in the oil and add the patties. Cook, turning once, until lightly browned and an instant-read meat thermometer inserted into the thickest part of one patty registers 145°F, 6 to 8 minutes in all.

MAKES 6 SERVINGS

RED LENTIL STEW

Bruce's revision of a North African recipe for the modern super-market uses a number of canned products, all of which can contain tons of sodium. A can of chickpeas or beans can have as much as 350 mg per serving (about 15 percent of the USDA's daily recommendation). The solution? Drain canned beans and legumes in a colander set in the sink, then rinse them well with cool water. And use a reduced-sodium broth, preferably a brand that's rich in real flavors—which will be brightened not with salt but with acid (in this case, lemon juice). Serve this aromatic main course over brown rice, steamed spinach, or even baked sweet potatoes.

1 tablespoon olive oil

1 large onion, chopped

2 large carrots, cut into ½-inch pieces

One 2½-pound medium kabocha squash, large butternut squash, or sugar pumpkin, peeled, seeded, and cut into 1-inch cubes (see Note)

1 quart reduced-sodium vegetable broth

1⅔ cups canned chickpeas, drained and rinsed (about one 15-ounce can)

1 cup red lentils

½ cup unsalted roasted peanuts, chopped

2 tablespoons reduced-sodium tomato paste

1 tablespoon minced peeled fresh ginger or jarred preminced ginger

1½ teaspoons ground cumin

½ teaspoon turmeric

½ teaspoon dried oregano

¼ teaspoon freshly ground black pepper

⅛ teaspoon saffron

¼ cup packed cilantro leaves

2 tablespoons lime juice

1. Heat a large saucepan or pot over medium heat, swirl in the oil, then add the onion, carrots, and squash. Stir over the heat until the onion begins to soften, about 4 minutes.

2. Pour in the broth, stir well, then add the chickpeas, lentils, peanuts, tomato paste, ginger, cumin, turmeric, oregano, pepper, and saffron. Bring to a full simmer.

3. Cover, reduce the heat to low, and simmer slowly until the vegetables are tender and the lentils have begun to break down, about 50 minutes.

4. Stir in the cilantro and lime juice just before serving.

Note: All hard, winter squashes are easiest to peel if they are first cut into chunks. Thin-skinned butternut squashes can be peeled with a vegetable peeler; thicker-skinned kabochas and pumpkins should have their rinds sliced off with a knife.

MAKES 6 SERVINGS

～～～～

GETTING THE MOST OUT OF EVERY GRAIN OF SALT

Prepared, processed, and packaged foods are doped with so much salt that it becomes the dominant taste. *And what taste is that?* we might ask. Honestly, does salt taste like anything on its own?

Yes, it does. It has a glorious flavor palette, derived from many minerals. But not run-of-the-mill table salt—which often begins as dense mineral clumps and is heated for sterilization, repeatedly washed of most accompanying minerals (many of which are also essential for good health like magnesium and potassium), and, finally, packed with silicate or sodium silicoaluminate to prevent clumping.

In the United States, table salt also has iodine in the mix (or more accurately, potassium iodine). In the 1920s, it was first added in to prevent goiters, a thyroid condition. But—one thing always leads to another, doesn't it?—dextrose, a sweetener, is added to stabilize the iodine.

Should we throw out common table salt? By no means. But we may want to use it more rarely, only in temperamental batters and doughs. Instead, we want types of salt that taste like something, that add real flavor to real food, such as the following:

Kosher Salt
It's not quite as refined as table salt and so has more mineral notes and aftertastes. Kosher salt is also coarser than refined table salt and thus a tad crunchier, a better coating for steaks on the grill, a rib

roast in the oven, or even make-your-own potato chips. However, it's not quite the ideal. That's . . .

Sea Salt
This salt has a higher mineral content, and thus a more complex taste. It comes in various grinds: *fine-grain* for sprinkling onto a dish when it's ready to eat or *coarse-grain* for adding to rubs, marinades, and coatings before any cooking happens.

Unrefined Sea Salt
It's only about 83 percent sodium chloride, chock-full of minerals like calcium, magnesium, iodine, and potassium. The taste is quite grown-up, sweet and minerally; the texture, not as crunchy as refined sea salt since it isn't dried in high-heat ovens.

And here are two Asian condiments that are prized for their pronounced, salty, sophisticated flavors:

Soy Sauce
It comes in several varieties, light to dark (not a reference to the sodium content but to how long it's aged after fermentation). They're all made from salted, fermented soy beans, a heady mix that runs the gamut from thin (so-called superior soy sauce) to viscous. In the end, Bruce often calls for reduced-sodium soy sauce in his recipes. Yes, it has a less complex taste. But it's being added over the heat, not drizzled as a condiment onto a dish, so complex flavors are volatilized and lost in the inferno of the wok or saucepan. If you're using soy sauce solely as a condiment at the table, consider the real deal, salty and with a distinct beany taste.

Fish Sauce
Sometimes called the ketchup of Southeast Asia, it's made from fermented fish parts, salt, and lots of aromatics. It has a pungent, acrid smell that mellows to a sweet/salty finish when heated. There are different varieties to explore: *nam pla* (the very heady Thai bottlings), *nuoc mam* (the slightly sweeter Vietnamese bottlings), and

fish gravy (the much milder Indonesian bottlings). You can buy fish sauce at almost all supermarkets these days, usually in the Asian aisle, although the selection at Asian grocers will be larger. Once the sauce is opened, store it in the refrigerator. If you have shellfish concerns, read the label carefully to choose a bottling made without shrimp or mollusks.

RECIPES THAT USE SALT FOR FLAVOR

From now on, don't use salt as an excuse for a lack of flavors. Instead, see it as the incredible, sophisticated enhancement it is. Choose one or both of the following recipes to prepare over the next few days. They're both real food, with a little salt but lots of flavor.

FISH FILLETS WITH TOMATOES, SHALLOTS, AND CREAM

Cream and salt are a natural combo—which is why they've been exploited so heavily. Still, we shouldn't run away just because this glorious pairing has been misused in the past. By eating real food, we can have it all!

½ cup unbleached all-purpose flour

1 teaspoon freshly ground black pepper

2 tablespoons unsalted butter, divided

Four 4- to 6-ounce thin white-flesh fish fillets, such as snapper, drum, or bass

1 large shallot, cut into thin slices, then minced into little bits

6 tablespoons dry white wine or dry vermouth (see Notes, page 28)

1¾ cups canned reduced-sodium diced tomatoes

2 tablespoons parsley leaves, chopped

2 tablespoons stemmed thyme leaves

¼ cup heavy cream

¼ to ½ teaspoon fine-grain sea salt

1. Use a fork to stir the flour and pepper on a dinner plate.

2. Melt 1 tablespoon of butter in a large skillet over medium heat.

3. Pat the fillets dry with paper towels; set them in the flour mixture, dredging them to coat both sides but shaking off any excess flour. Slip them into the skillet.

4. Cook until lightly browned, about 2 to 3 minutes. Flip and cook until lightly browned on the other side, about 1 to 2 minutes. The thin part of the fillet will pull into little flakes when gently scraped with a fork. Transfer to four serving plates or a serving platter; tent with foil to keep warm, if desired.

5. Melt the remaining 1 tablespoon of butter in the skillet, add the shallot, and cook, stirring frequently, until softened, about 1 minute.

6. Pour in the wine or vermouth, and bring to a simmer, scraping up any browned bits on the pan's bottom. Keep boiling until the liquid has turned into a thick glaze, about 2 minutes.

7. Add the canned tomatoes, parsley, and thyme. Continue simmering, stirring occasionally, until the sauce is thickened slightly and the tomatoes have broken down into a sauce, about 2 minutes.

8. Pour in the cream and bring back to a boil. Remove from the heat, stir in the salt, and spoon over the fillets.

MAKES 4 SERVINGS

CHICKEN LEGS ROASTED WITH GARLIC AND VEGETABLES

To serve this easy casserole, spoon the juicy drumsticks into individual bowls, then ladle the soupy vegetables and garlic cloves around them. As you eat the dish, squeeze the cloves out of their husks onto crusty bread, spreading the garlic like butter. By the way, the drumsticks are first skinned because they'll never get crispy in this covered casserole.

2 medium yellow onions, chopped

4 celery stalks, cut into ½-inch pieces

1 large butternut squash, halved lengthwise, seeded, peeled, and cut into ½-inch pieces

2 medium garlic heads, broken into individual cloves but not peeled

1 tablespoon olive oil, walnut oil, or unsalted butter, melted and cooled

2 tablespoons oregano leaves, minced, or 1 teaspoon dried oregano

2 teaspoons stemmed thyme or 1 teaspoon dried thyme

2 bay leaves

½ teaspoon freshly ground black pepper

12 skinless chicken drumsticks (see Note)

½ teaspoon fine-grain sea salt

1. Position a rack in the center of the oven and preheat to 350°F.

2. Mix the onion, celery, squash, garlic cloves, fat, oregano, and thyme in a large bowl; spread this mixture into a 9 x 13-inch baking pan or a large roasting pan, making a bed for the drumsticks. Wedge in the bay leaves, then season the mixture with pepper. Lay the drumsticks on top.

3. Cover and bake until the vegetables are soft and the drumsticks are cooked through, about 1 hour and 30 minutes. Let stand for 5 minutes at room temperature. Discard the bay leaves and sprinkle the dish with the salt just before serving.

Note: To skin a drumstick, grab the skin at the thick end and peel it back over the leg toward the thin end, pulling hard to get it off the last bit of knuckle. If it's too gross for you and skinned drumsticks aren't available at the supermarket, ask the butcher to do it for you.

MAKES 6 SERVINGS

The Second Detox: Fats

Many of us think fat is a toxin. Balderdash! Let's set the record straight:

✦ We need fats to thrive. Our brains use them to build essential neural structures.

✦ We need them to absorb essential nutrients. Vitamins A, D, E, and K are fat soluble; they can be brought into our bodies only via fat. So the next time you steam or roast some vitamin A-rich carrots, top them with a teaspoon or two of butter. Because you should!

✦ We need fats in order to sear, sauté, roast, and stir-fry. They let us raise the heat higher for longer, thereby breaking down sugars and proteins into complex flavors.

Chemically, fat is a subgroup of acids; culinarily, it's a densely-packed, low-moisture liquid or solid that brings great satisfaction. But nutritionally, fats come in two varieties: saturated and unsaturated. The difference has to do with the makeup of the fatty acids, the building blocks of all fats.

A fatty acid is like the letter E turned on its side, three little legs hanging down off a central line. That central line of the E is a sugar-like molecule; the three legs are dangling, chemical chains.

In a saturated fat, those dangling legs are stiff because the chemical bonds are linked up in perfect symmetry. A heavy hand with saturated fats is not good news for heart health.

By contrast, unsaturated fats are more wiggly. One or more of those legs hanging down has a less-than-secure bond. Monounsaturated fats have one bond in this flexible state—and so the molecules can slip by each other more easily. These fats tend to be liquid at room temperature but still become solid when chilled in the fridge. (Think olive oil or peanut oil.) Polyunsaturated fats have more than one flexible bond. These tend to be liquid even when they're in the fridge. (Think canola oil or almond oil.)

But here is the truth—and some good news: all fats and oils are a mixed bag, containing saturated, monounsaturated, and polyunsaturated fats. We call butter a saturated fat because it has more saturated fat than the other two kinds. But it definitely has all three. And it definitely brings a lot of satisfaction to a piece of toast!

NOW THE BAD NEWS

We eat too many fats—not because they're rich and satisfying, but because:

✦ They're in copious supply, dumped willy-nilly into packaged, prepared, and processed foods.

Starting to see a pattern here? We need something and are rewarded internally for finding it, but then are given so much that we lose that pleasure response altogether.

Consider packaged cookies. They're loaded with fat because they have to stay moist on the shelf long enough for someone to pick them up and think they taste good.

Ever made cookies at home? Ever had them sit around for, oh, a month? If they don't mold, they'll probably be rocks (or moldy rocks). But not those packaged ones.

Then one thing leads to another. (And another pattern, eh?) Fats go rancid over time, so adding more requires more stabilizers, preservatives, and emulsifiers. More fat, more fake.

✦ Most of those overused fats are utterly tasteless.

Why do people butter their bread? Or dip it in olive oil? Because it tastes good. You'll never see anyone corn-oiling their bread. You have to taste a fat to get any satisfaction from it.

Think about most run-of-the-mill bagged potato chips. They're fried in an utterly flavorless oil—and lots of it, to boot. Do you even know the oil used? Probably not. Yet you may be eating lots.

Now contrast those chips with the ones we made when we were experimenting with salt, the ones oven-fried in olive oil to give them a savory flavor (see page 118). We used way less oil and got way more flavor.

Or what about bottled salad dressings? They're a major source of fat, about 8 to 15 grams for a measly 2 tablespoon serving. But most of their fats are no more than a slick bit of tastelessness on the plate. Our salad dressings are stocked with big, bold oils for better taste (see page 68).

Even when you cook at home, you might be tempted to use flavorless fats. Check your pantry. What's on hand? Probably bottles of tasteless oils as well as some sort of solid vegetable shortening.

No wonder we eat more. We're so unsatisfied.

But before things can get better, they're about to get worse.

WHEN FAT CEASES TO BE REAL FOOD

These days, most fats are processed or modified in some way—extracted under heat high enough to destroy nutrition, refined with all sorts of solvents, and/or made from genetically modified this-and-that.

Why? Well, first there's cost. Because of their seemingly eternal shelf life, highly refined fats are cheap, despite the more complicated processes to make them.

And then there's their neutral flavor. Less taste appeals to more people. Or so the marketing theory goes.

Consider canola oil, made from Canadian rapeseeds, a high-yield grass crop (the name canola is derived from *Canadian oil*). The little seeds are quite nutritious with a monounsaturated fat content (like olive oil) of 57 percent and at least 10 percent omega-3 fatty acids, the heart-healthy stuff in walnuts and salmon. However, these good factors also give the oil almost no shelf life: it goes rancid. So it's often processed. Into oblivion. The oil is taken from the seeds via high-heat mechanized processing and chemical solvents. It's then further refined, bleached, and degummed. Unfortunately, those omega-3s go rancid during the high-heat processing, leaving foul odors in the oil. So it also has to undergo chemical deodorization before it's bottled. That's a lot of work to turn a pretty good fat into a tasteless, shelf-stable one. (That said, there are cold-pressed canola oils on the market. We'll get to the difference in a minute; but as always, read those labels!)

Some modern, manufactured fats are not only tasteless but downright dangerous—that is, trans fats, made by beating hydrogen into oils, in a misguided attempt to make them solid at room temperature and thus more shelf-stable. A can of hydrogenated shortening can last in your pantry for a year or more, while the cold-pressed oil will go rancid in a few months, if not weeks.

Those trade-offs are not worth it. Bruce and I place all industrially hydrogenated oils in the category of *not real food*. Trans fats have been blamed for raising blood cholesterol and a bevy of health problems. As Marion Nestle, professor of Nutrition, Food Studies, and Public Health at New York University, puts it, "[I]f you can avoid trans fats, you should. These fatty acids may be only a small part of your total dietary fat, but small changes in your diet can add up to significant health benefits, and this one change is well worth making."[6]

But forget about any health claims for a second. After all, we're mostly concerned about taste—and therefore, pleasure. Which just doesn't exist with those processed fats. So we're encouraged to eat more because we get less, because we lack the basic signals of satiety that flavor brings.

FLAVOR FIRST AND FOREMOST

We need to detox from the slather. Here's our general rule:

✦ Always use a fat or oil to enhance flavor.

One warning: watch the heat. Highly refined oils can take punishing heat better than flavorful oils—which can ignite! If a pan or pot is smoking hot, don't add a flavorful oil or fat. Pull the cookware off the heat, let it cool down, and start again. Yes, you want some sizzle when you add the onion, but you don't want the oil to flash into a fire.

We also have a follow-up to our rule:

✦ Substitute a flavorful oil in any recipe that calls for a less-flavorful one.

If a recipe calls for canola oil to cook a pork chop, consider replacing it with walnut oil for more flavor. If a recipe for chili calls for safflower oil, substitute butter.

Many people are using olive oil these days, popularized by a gaggle of celebrity chefs. We can't agree more with the trend. There's no doubt that olive oil adds loads of flavor. But not all olive oils are created equal. A cheap, flavorless olive oil is little better than any other tasteless oil in cueing satisfaction. However, don't waste expensive extra-virgin olive oil in a two-hour pot of soup. A sturdy but still flavorful olive oil, sold in bulk in large cans, will do the trick every time.

Finally, we've got a second follow-up to our rule:

✦ Because a flavorful oil packs a bigger punch, half the quantity of oil called for in standard recipes.

Just be wary of baking. You can't cut down the fat or oil in a brownie or cookie recipe at will. But you can definitely replace a less flavorful oil with a more flavorful one (like pecan or walnut oil) in equal measure.

So let's get to cooking with more flavor. Try your hand at these recipes and watch how a bold bit of oil changes everything!

RED PEPPER HUMMUS

Bruce's version of the classic Middle Eastern dip includes a roasted red pepper for even more flavor, a good canvas for a full-flavored oil. Make a simple lunch out of a serving with some cut-up veggies and a toasted whole wheat pita—or the salad recipe that follows.

1¾ cups canned chickpeas, drained and rinsed

1 large jarred roasted red pepper or pimiento, rinsed

2 medium garlic cloves, minced

¼ cup lemon juice

¼ cup tahini (see Note)

½ teaspoon freshly ground black pepper

¼ teaspoon kosher salt or sea salt

1 tablespoon toasted sesame oil, pumpkin seed oil, or toasted walnut oil

1. Place the chickpeas, roasted red pepper, garlic, lemon juice, tahini, pepper, and salt in a food processor fitted with the chopping blade. Process until smooth, scraping down the insides of the canister a couple times to make sure everything takes a death spiral onto the blades.

2. Scrape the puree into a bowl; drizzle the oil on top. If you want to make the dip ahead of time, don't add the oil; instead, cover and refrigerate the hummus for up to 3 days, drizzling with the oil when you're ready to serve it.

Note: Tahini is a paste made from toasted sesame seeds, sort of like a sesame-seed version of peanut butter. Once opened, store tahini in the refrigerator, covered, for up to 9 months.

MAKES 4 SERVINGS

SESAME CARROT SALAD

This dish has got it all: great chew, great flavors, and lots of real food! Paired with the Red Pepper Hummus, it's a satisfying meal.

1 pound carrots, grated through the large holes of a box grater

2 tablespoons rice vinegar (see Note, page 114)

1 tablespoon toasted sesame oil

2 teaspoons minced peeled fresh ginger or jarred preminced ginger

½ teaspoon fine-grain sea salt

Mix all the ingredients in a large bowl. Serve at once or store, covered, in the fridge for up to 3 days.

MAKES 4 SERVINGS

GRILLED FENNEL WITH AVOCADO OIL

Once again, a little drizzle of a flavorful oil makes a simple dish extraordinary. Consider serving this with some rotisseried chicken you picked up at the supermarket.

2 fennel bulbs

1 tablespoon avocado oil

½ teaspoon freshly ground black pepper

¼ teaspoon kosher salt or fine-grain sea salt

1. Trim and discard the fennel fronds by cutting off the stalks that may come out of the top of the bulb. Also trim off any feathery fronds. If rusted or brown, peel off the outer layer of the bulb. Slice the bulb into ½-inch-thick slices through the root.

2. Heat a grill to high heat or a grill pan over medium-high heat until smoking. Set the fennel on the grill directly over the heat or in the pan and cook until lightly browned on each side, about 6 minutes, turning once.

3. Transfer to a serving plate, drizzle with the oil, and sprinkle with the pepper and salt.

MAKES 2 SERVINGS (CAN BE DOUBLED OR TRIPLED)

OLIVE OIL COOKIES

Better oils make better desserts! These Italian wonders deserve the best olive oil you can muster. They're made with semolina flour, a particularly coarse flour made from durum wheat. Look for it at specialty Italian stores, all gourmet stores, and online suppliers.

⅓ cup sugar

1 large egg

2 tablespoons plus 2½ teaspoons extra-virgin olive oil

¼ teaspoon salt

1½ cups unbleached all-purpose flour

⅓ cup semolina flour

½ tablespoon finely grated orange zest

1 teaspoon baking powder

1. Position a rack in the center of the oven and preheat to 350°F.

2. Whisk the sugar, egg, olive oil, and salt in a large bowl until smooth.

3. Stir in both flours, the orange zest, and baking powder just until a dry batter forms.

4. Shape this mixture into a log about 5 inches long and 3 inches thick. Set it on a baking sheet and bake for 30 minutes.

5. Cool the log on the baking sheet for 1 hour. Meanwhile, reduce the oven temperature to 325°F.

6. Transfer the log to a cutting board and slice into ½-inch rounds. Set these on the baking sheet and bake for 20 minutes, turning once halfway through baking to make sure both sides get crisp against the hot baking sheet.

MAKES 10 COOKIES

FAT 201: A DIFFERENTIATION AMONG KINDS

When we talk about *fat*, we sometimes mean a generic category. *Add the fat when the skillet is hot*—as if butter or olive oil were the same thing. They're not.

There are actually two different types of fat:

1. Fats Derived from Plants

These are technically oils, liquid at room temperature and derived from fruits (i.e., olives or coconuts), seeds (i.e., sunflower or sesame seeds), or nuts (i.e., pecans, almonds, walnuts, or hazelnuts).

Almost every oil has the same number of calories: 120 per tablespoon. So if a tasteless oil has the same number of calories as a tasty one, why would anyone settle for less flavor?

The answer is cost. Flavorful oils are undoubtedly expensive. However, you can sometimes buy bulk tins, provided the containers are indeed made of metal, not glass (light makes most flavorful oils go rancid more quickly).

But the good news is that you'll be using less, so the cost will be prolonged over their use. Also look for them at specialty supermarkets: Indian, Asian, and Latin American, for example. The prices are often much better. And look for Internet suppliers—or coupons online.

Here are the basic choices:

	WHAT?	WHEN?	ANYTHING ELSE?
Avocado oil	An emerald green oil with a luxurious but light avocado taste	Great for sautéing (scallops, chicken); excellent as a base in chile-laced dishes; also a flavorful condiment drizzled over vegetables	Since avocados are technically berries, this is the only common berry oil
Nut oils: almond, hazelnut, pecan, pistachio, and walnut	There are basically two types: those made from untoasted nuts (sweet, pale, and perfumy) and those made from toasted nuts (dark, heavy, and sophisticated)	Untoasted oils: for cooking—as a base for sautés, braises, and stews, as well as the oil in batters and doughs. Toasted versions: as a condiment, drizzle on steamed, grilled, or roasted foods	We like untoasted almond or pecan oil for cooking and toasted walnut or hazelnut oil as a condiment
Olive oil	A bright, almost refreshing flavor, an excellent go-to oil for the modern kitchen	For sautéing, braising, grilling, and roasting. Better-quality bottlings are great as bread dips or salad oils	Keep a sturdy, aromatic, standard olive oil for cooking and a delicate, more expensive one for a condiment— like a drizzle on mashed potatoes with lots of cracked black pepper. The better the oil, the less it should be heated

	WHAT?	WHEN?	ANYTHING ELSE?
Peanut oil	A mild peanut flavor that can become assertive in some Asian bottlings	As the base of many stir-fries as well as for simple sautés, oven-frying, roasting, and grilling	Refined bottlings lose much of their peanuty flavor; unrefined bottlings are far tastier but may ignite over excessive heat
Pumpkin seed oil	A dark green to black oil, highly flavorful with a toasty taste	Only as a condiment—tossed with warm pasta and shaved Parmesan, or drizzled onto bean dips	Because it's expensive, some manufacturers cut it with tasteless oils like sunflower oil. Read the labels to get the real thing
Sesame oil	A full-flavored oil with a sophisticated finish and a taste like tahini. There are both toasted and untoasted versions	The untoasted version: as a base for stir-fries, curries, and other strongly flavored dishes, particularly with Asian flavorings. The toasted version: as a condiment, lightly drizzled over finished stir-fries or used in salad dressings	Sesame oil has a strong, assertive taste—use it sparingly until you get the hang of it

These five tips will make the most out of your oils:

1. Look for words like *first cold-pressed* or *cold pressed* (the latter meaning it's a slightly less tasty oil, not necessarily made from the first time the fruit or nuts were pressed).

2. Avoid any oil that marks itself as *refined* (as in *from refined olives*). The oil may have been extracted using industrial solvents. If so, it's not real food.

3. When you first open a flavorful oil, it should smell bright and clean, about like the fruit, plant, or seed from which it was derived. If it smells acrid or rancid, return it for full credit.

4. To preserve freshness, store flavorful oils, once opened, in the refrigerator. Some may cloud or solidify. They will return to their liquid state within a few minutes out of the fridge.

5. All flavorful oils taste best at room temperature. You have to get the walnut oil out of the fridge for ten minutes before you drizzle it on roasted veggies. If you forget, do what Bruce does: run the bottle under warm tap water until there's enough liquefied oil for your needs.

2. Fats Derived from Animals

These are indeed technically *fats*—by which we mean *mammal* or *bird fats*, from pigs, cows, sheep, goats, chickens, ducks, geese, or what have you. Butter and the like tend to be solid (or close to it) at room temperature.

These fats have different calorie amounts, all *fewer* than those in oil partly because oils are denser and because fats often have other solids in the mix. For example, butter contains both dairy fat *and* residual milk solids—that is, the white bits floating in the yellow fat of melted butter.

That said, we shouldn't chow down willy-nilly on fats because we can save a few calories. For one thing, the savings aren't all that dramatic. And all animal fats contain varying amounts of saturated fat, which, as we said, may lead to some health problems. While animal fats are definitely real food, they should be handled with the delicate touch they so richly deserve. You don't need ½ cup of duck fat in a recipe—but boy, will a tablespoon as the base of a chicken breast sauté make all the difference in the world!

Here are the basic choices:

	WHAT?	WHEN?	ANYTHING ELSE?
Butter	A churned fat from milk (not just cow, but also goat, sheep, yak, and even horse in some parts of the world)	Use for everything from baking and sautéing to a condiment spread	Unsalted remains the culinary standard. Cultured butter is made with various bacteria, much as yogurt, and has slightly sour undertones
Lard	Made from rendered pig fat, with a silky, delicate taste	It makes incredibly crisp cookies and is great to spread on the baking sheet for oven-frying	Rendered bacon fat is a spectacular, smoky version of this fat, used as a base for savory braises and stews
Duck or goose fat	A luxurious fat, smooth and quite sophisticated	For sautéing or roasting—although some in southern France have been known to use it as a condiment on cooked veggies (like butter)	A little goes a very long way
Schmaltz (a.k.a. chicken fat)	A creamy, delicate fat, best in small doses	Of all the flavorful fats, it's the most neutral (although barely). Use it as a base for soups and stews	Your great-grandmother would be so pleased!

When you're cooking with an animal fat, take into account where it comes from—not what animal, but what environment. Lard from organic, pasture-raised pigs is basically a monounsaturated fat, sort of like olive oil. But the unrefrigerated lard sold in solid blocks at the supermarket has been hydrogenated for shelf life, turned from a luxury product into an industrial fat. To find good lard, ask for it at the butcher case of high-end supermarkets or develop a connection to a local farm, perhaps at a farmers' market.

Any fat may contain traces of whatever the animal has eaten. While there's little cause for panic, here are three steps you can take to have better quality, real fats:

1. Buy better-quality animal fats.

2. Check out producers, to see what their specific practices are.

3. Investigate organic fats. If you're ever going to go organic, fats are the first place to start.

Finally, there's one exception to our two categories: fish oils. Although these are derived from animals (salmon or cod, for example), they are lumped with the other oils for chemical reasons. That said, fish oils are *not* culinary fats. No recipe will ever ask us to add 1 tablespoon salmon oil to a skillet—mostly because it's so stinky.

BETTER OILS AND FATS MAKE FOR BETTER MEALS

More flavor is better than less, and a little bit of better beats a lot of worse any day! So use oils and fats to good effect. Bruce has cut down the amount in each recipe, the better to let the natural flavors come through—and also to relish the oil or fat used!

NO-FRY EGGPLANT PARMESAN CASSEROLE

First off, Bruce revamped the classic by taking out so much of the otherwise tasteless oil (used to deep-fry the eggplant disks). Then he simplified the flavors, the better to let that olive oil shine.

1 tablespoon olive oil, plus a little
   more for oiling the baking sheets
2 medium onions, finely chopped
4 medium garlic cloves, minced
1 tablespoon minced oregano or
   2 teaspoons dried oregano
1 tablespoon stemmed thyme or
   2 teaspoons dried thyme
7½ cups reduced-sodium diced
   tomatoes (two 28-ounce cans)

2 bay leaves
¼ teaspoon grated nutmeg
2 teaspoons kosher salt or fine-grain
   sea salt
2 medium eggplants, sliced into
   ½-inch-thick disks
6 ounces Parmigiano-Reggiano,
   shaved into thin strips with a
   vegetable peeler or a sharp knife

1. Heat a medium saucepan over medium heat. Pour in the oil, then add the onion and cook until soft, about 3 minutes, stirring frequently.

2. Drop in the garlic, oregano, and thyme. Cook until aromatic, about 10 seconds.

3. Pour in the tomatoes, add the bay leaves and nutmeg, then bring the sauce to a simmer.

4. Reduce the heat to low, and simmer, uncovered, until thickened, about 20 minutes, to create a wet sauce, not too thick, but also not soupy.

5. Meanwhile, lightly salt the eggplant slices on both sides and lay them out on paper towels on the counter to sweat for 15 minutes. Position the racks in the top and bottom thirds of the oven and preheat to 375°F.

6. Blot the eggplant dry with paper towels. This will not only dry them but also remove some of the salt. Lightly oil two lipped baking sheets with a little olive oil on a crumpled paper towel. Lay the eggplant slices evenly and in one layer across the sheets. Place one tray on each rack and bake for 10 minutes. Turn the slices over, then reverse the baking trays top to bottom. Continue baking until the slices are a little dried out and beginning to soften, about 10 more minutes. After you remove them from the oven, lower the top rack so that it's in the middle of the oven and maintain the oven's temperature.

7. Spoon about 1 cup of the tomato sauce into a 9 x 13-inch baking dish. Lay half the eggplant slices in the dish, making a layer. Top them with half the shaved cheese. Spoon and spread about 1½ cups tomato sauce over the cheese. Place the remaining eggplant slices in the pan as a single layer, then place the remaining cheese on top of them. Spoon the remaining tomato sauce over the casserole.

8. Bake in the middle of the oven until bubbling, about 25 minutes. Let stand at room temperature for 5 minutes before serving.

MAKES 8 SERVINGS

SPLIT PEA SOUP

Split peas, a variety grown to be dried and halved along a natural seam, don't require presoaking; instead, they slowly melt over the heat into a luxurious soup. They're so starchy, they almost seem to buzz when a flavorful oil is used as a condiment.

8 cups (2 quarts) reduced-sodium
    vegetable broth

2 cups green split peas, picked over
    for tiny stones and rinsed

1½ cups water

1 medium yellow onion, chopped

8 ounces Canadian bacon, diced

1 tablespoon finely minced lemon zest

2 medium carrots, thinly sliced

2 medium celery stalks, thinly sliced

¼ cup dill fronds, minced

½ teaspoon freshly ground black
    pepper

1 tablespoon lemon juice

Avocado oil, a toasted nut oil, or
    toasted sesame oil, as garnish

1. Bring the broth, split peas, water, onion, Canadian bacon, and lemon zest to a simmer in a large pot over medium-high heat. Reduce heat and simmer slowly, uncovered, for 1 hour, stirring occasionally.

2. Stir in the carrots, celery, dill, and pepper. Cover and simmer slowly until the vegetables are tender, about 45 minutes, stirring occasionally.

3. Stir in the lemon juice before serving. Then drizzle about 1 teaspoon avocado oil or other oil over each bowlful at the table. There's no salt in the dish because the Canadian bacon is salty by nature. If you'd like more, taste it first and then sprinkle a few grains of sea salt over your serving.

MAKES 6 SERVINGS

CRAB CAKES

Nothing enhances the flavor of crab like butter! Pasteurized crabmeat is a boon to home cooks—you don't have to spend hours picking the meat out of the shells. It's readily available in the refrigerator case of your supermarket, usually near the fish counter. No need to use jumbo lump or even lump, an unnecessary expense in this recipe. Serve these crab cakes atop a lemon-juice–dressed salad of greens, radish sprouts, and sliced peaches.

1 pound crabmeat, picked over for any bits of cartilage and shell

½ cup whole wheat panko bread crumbs (see Note)

¼ cup low-fat mayonnaise

1 tablespoon minced chives or the green part of a scallion

1 tablespoon Dijon mustard

1 teaspoon celery seed

½ teaspoon lemon juice

¼ teaspoon freshly ground black pepper

Several dashes hot red pepper sauce, like Tabasco sauce, to taste

1 tablespoon unsalted butter

1. Mix the crab, bread crumbs, mayonnaise, chives, mustard, celery seed, lemon juice, pepper, and Tabasco sauce in a large bowl; form into four patties.

2. Melt the butter in a large skillet over medium heat. Slip the patties into the pan and cook for 3 minutes. Turn and cook until golden, about 3 more minutes.

Note: Panko bread crumbs are a Japanese specialty, a form of dried bread crumbs now widely available in the United States. They're coarse and have a great crunch. (The English name, in fact, is a redundancy since *panko* means "bread crumbs" in Japanese.) And as for that low-fat mayonnaise, read the labels to make sure you're getting the real thing, with nothing fake in the mix.

MAKES 4 CRAB CAKES

CHICKEN, FENNEL, AND MUSHROOM CASSEROLE

Mushrooms offer an earthy, autumnal punch to this cool-day dinner. Although it tastes great hot from the oven, the fennel and mushroom combination mellows beautifully overnight. Serve it over cooked whole wheat pasta, brown rice, or wilted greens.

2 tablespoons unsalted butter, duck fat, or goose fat

6 boneless, skinless chicken thighs (about 1½ pounds)

1 medium yellow onion, halved and cut into thin rings

1 small green bell pepper, stemmed, seeded, and diced (see Note, page 5)

1 small fennel bulb (about ½ pound), trimmed of any fronds or stems, any brown bits removed, the bulb then halved and thinly sliced

4 ounces (¼ pound) cremini or white button mushrooms, sliced

2 garlic cloves, minced

2 teaspoons rosemary or oregano leaves, minced

1 teaspoon finely grated orange zest

2 tablespoons white wine vinegar

¾ cup reduced-sodium, fat-free chicken broth

1 tablespoon reduced-sodium tomato paste

½ teaspoon kosher salt or fine-grain sea salt

1. Position a rack in the center of the oven and preheat to 350°F.

2. Melt the butter in a large, high-sided skillet over medium heat. Add the chicken thighs and brown on all sides, turning occasionally, about 4 minutes. Transfer to a 9-inch square baking dish.

3. Add the onion and bell pepper to the skillet; cook, stirring often, until soft, about 3 minutes.

4. Stir in the fennel; continue cooking, stirring often, until somewhat softened at the edges, about 2 minutes.

5. Add the mushrooms, garlic, rosemary or oregano, and orange zest. Cook, stirring occasionally, until the mushrooms give off their internal liquid, it comes to a simmer, and reduces to a thick glaze, about 4 minutes.

6. Pour in the vinegar, scraping up any browned bits on the pan's bottom.

7. Stir in the broth, tomato paste, and salt. Bring to a simmer, then pour over the thighs.

8. Cover the dish with foil and bake until bubbling, about 45 minutes. Cool 10 minutes before serving.

MAKES 6 SERVINGS

~~~~~~

</div>

The Third Detox: Sugars

Let's start by celebrating how incredible sweet things can be with this straightforward, Mediterranean dessert, perfect for an evening treat or a weekend breakfast. Taste it carefully, making sure to savor the flavors in all the ways you've learned.

<div align="center">

CLAFOUTI

</div>

A clafouti is made by baking fruit in a thickened custard (usually cherries, but there's no reason to stand on ceremony). Bruce's is sweetened with honey for a rich dessert that needs no other fandango.

Unsalted butter for greasing the baking dish

8 ripe apricots, halved and pitted; or 8 ripe figs, stemmed and halved; or about 30 Bing cherries, stemmed, halved, and pitted

4 large egg yolks, at room temperature

¾ cup low-fat sour cream (do not use fat-free)

⅓ cup honey

¼ cup low-fat milk

2 teaspoons vanilla extract

¼ teaspoon salt

½ cup unbleached all-purpose flour

1. Position a rack in the center of the oven and preheat to 400°F.

2. Lightly butter a 9-inch square pan. Lay the fruit cut side up across the bottom of the pan.

3. Whisk the egg yolks, sour cream, honey, milk, vanilla, and salt in a large bowl until smooth. Whisk in the flour until smooth. Gently scrape and pour the mixture over the fruit in the prepared pan, taking care not to dislodge them.

4. Bake until lightly browned and a knife inserted into the custard without its touching a piece of fruit comes out clean, about 25 minutes. Cool on a wire rack for 15 minutes before scooping up to serve, or cover and store in the refrigerator for up to 2 days.

MAKES 6 SERVINGS

~~~~~~

THE SWEETENING OF AMERICA

Ah, that clafouti. It's one of the many reasons Bruce and I love sweets. If Dr. Atkins hated it, we're all for it.

But we've always considered these things treats. Which means we're often disappointed—even when we're trying to make better choices. Almost everything in the organic section of our supermarket is a sweet snack of some kind, if not a sweetened breakfast cereal: cane syrup this and brown sugar that. Does everything have to be cloying, sticky, or syrupy all the time?

Apparently so. By 2003, Americans were eating 142 *pounds* of various sweeteners *per person per year*.[7] That's the equivalent of about 16,000 teaspoons of table sugar—or just shy of *1 cup per day*![8]

The United States is one of the world's largest producers of sugar and sweeteners *and* one of the largest importers.[9] We can't make enough to keep up with the demand—and the increasing use of corn syrup and its manufactured derivatives shows no sign of stopping.

Here's what the USDA has to say about the matter: "[S]ugar is the number one food additive. It turns up in some unlikely places, such as pizza, bread, hot dogs, boxed mixed rice, soup, crackers, spaghetti sauce, lunch meat, canned vegetables, fruit drinks, flavored yogurt, ketchup, salad dressing, mayonnaise, and some peanut butter."[10]

It's a myth to say that sugar is bad for us. Despite anecdotal evidence, it doesn't make us hyperactive. Yes, mothers at a birthday party will swear that the cake sent their children over the edge, but controlled studies have failed to find a link between kids running amuck and sugar intake.

But this much is true: something sweet should be enjoyed for what it is. It's not a snack midafternoon. It's not a reward for dieting all day. It's a pleasure, part of a rounded set of food choices.

NEEDING IT, GETTING IT

We're hardwired for the sweet stuff. Glucose, one of the simplest sugars, sustains life in almost all organisms on this planet. It's the basic energy of cells. Almost every carb we ingest (from bread to chocolate candy, pasta to fruit juice) is broken down into glucose, which is stored in our livers and muscles, then distributed as we go about our daily activities, from knitting to exercising, gardening to sleeping.

Even as you read these very words, you're burning glucose. Our brains run on the stuff. Without it, we become sluggish, our mental processes impaired.[11]

The body is all about efficiency. Eat a piece of candy and it's a quick-step dance to glucose in the digestive track and then in the brain, way easier and more readily available than the slower, waltzing, complex carbs found in other foods. So we get an instant reward for finding a quick way to feed our brains.

It starts early on. Infants go for the sweet. There are sticky compounds in our mothers' milk that cause us to nurse almost immediately.

In fact, babies will regulate their intake of water based on their needs—until sucrose (or table sugar) is added. Then they'll continue to swallow the solution beyond what they need in order to stay healthy.[12]

But glucose isn't water. As adults, we sweat, we dehydrate, and we need water right away. By contrast, glucose is stored a couple days for when it's needed. Healthy people don't shed excess glucose. Although we need it to function, we don't need as much as we're getting. We've become little sugar banks.

Once, sugars were difficult to consume. Fruits and some vegetables, the main sources, weren't available year-round. In fact, that need for sugars may explain the rise of the craft of baking: breads, rice pastries, and corn cakes are a way to preserve a rich source of carbohydrates (and thus, slower, waltzing sugars, but sugars nonetheless).

These days, there's no shortage. Modern marketing is all about taking that biological dictate, the need for the sweet stuff, and pushing it into overdrive, offering us sugar at every turn, until we're practically addled.

As Dr. Barbara J. Rolls put it to me, "We're so overexposed to the stuff that it's simply become a part of our eating repertoire." She demurred when I asked her about whether we're addicted to sugars and simply said that "people have the best intentions" but find themselves hemmed in by bad choices. Sugars, particularly the ones found in high-calorie foods, like ketchup or cinnamon buns, have become expected, even the norm. "It's really hard to break established behaviors," she concluded.[13]

So let's step back from what's become the norm to make clear what our choices are—all in an effort to get the sweet stuff back to its rightful position: a small, pleasurable part of a well-rounded set of choices.

To do that, let's start out by examining what's definitely not real food and work our way across our real food chart, ferreting out the important points to find real pleasure.

NOT REAL SWEETENERS

Chemical Fake-Out Sweeteners

One of the persistent answers to our excessive sugar consumption has been to offer various chemical substitutes that rob sweets of any calories, thereby supposedly making the abundant supply benign. Drink a soda without gaining weight! Eat a cookie without putting on the pounds! Bake a cake that's not (so) bad for you! Many a diet plan is simply a matter of demonizing sugar and replacing it with the fake stuff.

As we've already discussed, ongoing research suggests that artificially sweetened products fake out the brain, stimulating it to expect a big calorie hit—which then never materializes, leaving us in the lurch and searching for those calories (see pages 41–42).

No one is saying these chemical sweeteners are necessarily dangerous to our health in and of themselves. The FDA has tested each and approved limits on consumption that almost defy logic. But there's a problem with faking ourselves out. We think we're getting something for nothing. We've all opened a box of reduced- or no-sugar treats and eaten way more than the suggested serving size because . . . well, we didn't even think about it. Maybe we thought we could; maybe we thought that by buying the reduced-sugar product we were doing ourselves a favor. Then we looked at the label only to discover that we didn't really save that many calories at all.

Look at this comparison:

	SERVING SIZE	CALORIES	CARBS
Nabisco Oreo Sandwich Cookies Golden Original	35 grams	170	25 g
Nabisco SnackWells Lemon Cream Sugar-Free Sandwich Cookies	32 grams	130	23 g

At the store, we might be tempted to pick up the SnackWells because they will save us a bunch of calories since they're sugar-free. But regular and sugar-free cookies are often similar in carbs, often even comparable in calories. Plus, in our example the serving size of the sugar-free cookies is slightly less. And beyond all that, 40 calories will not change the world, no matter how much we want it to. And besides, we're often tempted to eat more than the suggested amount because we think we can—or because we missed the cues to satiety a real sweetener can bring.

In truth, fat, sugar, and salt are in such a symbiotic relationship in our world that when one is lowered, the others may well be increased to compensate: less fat, more sugar and salt; less sugar, more fat and salt; less salt, more sugar (and probably fat).

Plus, when the sugar is taken out of a product, chemical preservatives and additives are often poured in to aid its texture and keep it on the shelf longer.

Our journey is about returning to food that tastes better, food that has spent less time in a chemical lab or a manufacturing plant, food that pleases in healthy ways, the better to cue satiety. Fake sweeteners just don't fit the bill.

High-Fructose Corn Syrup
Corn syrup has a telling history. It's a basic sugar, made from cornstarch, the white, snowy stuff we can buy in a box at the supermarket.

Ever tasted it? Cornstarch is surprisingly neutral, hardly sweet at all, maybe just a tad on the back of the tongue, like milled flour. To become corn syrup, it's treated with enzymes that snap the molecules down into glucose and a few leftovers. The powdery starch becomes the viscous liquid found in those bottles in the baking aisle (to which, by the way, salt and vanilla have been added). *Now* it's sweet. Wow.

But apparently not sweet enough for many of us. In the end, glucose isn't the sweetest natural sugar out there. That's fructose, about two and a half times sweeter. It really stimulates our taste, probably because our tongues don't know the difference between one type of sugar and another.

Which is one of the reasons industrial food chemists are keen on getting really sweet stuff into what we eat. We want more, we buy more.

By doping that same corn syrup with more enzymes, some of that glucose—up to 55 percent—can be snapped down into fructose, thus creating various strains of *high-fructose corn syrup*.[14]

Remember that bit about how living cells need glucose to thrive? They don't need much fructose. So high-fructose corn syrup is a preservative in ways that glucose isn't. All things, down to tiny bacteria, want to have a go at glucose. Fructose? Not so much.

What's more, it's cheap. After all, if you can put something that's lots sweeter into your product, you need to use lots less. Costs go down; shareholders are happy. So high-fructose corn syrup has gone into thousands of things. In 2008, the United States produced 18,148,000 pounds.[15] Naturally, since we're eating so much, it's been blamed for a range of health problems, including the obesity epidemic.

In the end, portion size and calorie count are to blame for our weight gain. But high-fructose corn syrup has been at the center of that problem: a calorie-rich sweetener, often a partner to industrial fats, all heavily refined, all made in a chemical lab, cheap enough that they can be tossed into big-portion meals, to be made even sweeter (and fattier) without much added cost.

To relearn the pleasure of food and lose weight, we have to cleanse our palates of the things that have driven food into a sticky-sweet realm. We have to get back to appreciating sweet for what it is: a wonderful indulgence. High-fructose corn syrup doesn't fit the bill.

BARELY REAL SWEETENERS

In this category, we'll put things that are less refined (some only slightly less) but nonetheless still sweet. Here, we'll find:

✦ **Refined white sugar**, made by pressing sugarcane, beets, date palms, or sorghum to extract their juices. Through a variety of processes, the juice is treated with alkalis to remove impurities and neutralize its taste. It's then subjected to a host of processes including boiling, skimming, cooling, filtering, separating, sieving, and/or vacuum-thickening in various centrifuges and chambers. The molasses is removed and at long last, the result is the pure white stuff we know as *refined white sugar*—or more commonly, *table sugar*.[16]

✦ **Brown sugar**, made by adding some of the extracted, natural molasses back to refined sugar. Therefore, it's not somehow healthier or more natural than refined sugar—it's just refined sugar with something that was taken out put back in. The difference between light and dark brown sugar is simply the amount of added molasses (more for dark).

✦ **Corn syrup**, a glucose solution from cornstarch, one we've already met (see High-Fructose Corn Syrup, page 155). But don't be fooled by light corn syrup. We were once on a national TV show and added some light corn syrup to a batter. The host immediately said, "Oh, light. We like that." Neither Bruce nor I had the guts to correct her on air, but *light* has nothing to do with calories. *Light* is a moniker to place it in opposition to *dark* corn syrup, which includes caramel coloring. The difference between the two simply affects the color of the candy or baked good.

✦ **Molasses**, often made as a by-product of sugar refining. The initial straining results in a somewhat lighter molasses, still quite complex in its taste, often used in baking for brownies, cookies, and such. Further boilings create even more intense tastes, like the famed blackstrap molasses, a triple-boiled-down product that is actually less sweet and quite mineral rich—definitely an acquired taste. There are brands of natural, unsulfured molasses, less processed and probably more in the *almost real food* category.

✦ **Rice syrup**, one in a long line of sweetening products with quasi-health claims. Sometimes called brown rice syrup, it's made through a similar process as corn syrup: rice cooked with enzymes. Be wary: sweet is sweet; calories are calories. And rice syrup is a tasteless sweetener, adding little satisfaction to a final dish, about the way the rest of these sweeteners in this category do.

✦ **Fruit syrups and sweeteners**—tastier perhaps, but nonetheless refined and reconstituted, exceptionally sweet. When a product claims to be made with *100 percent fruit*, read the label. If it includes fruit concentrates, it basically includes straight-on, extracted sweeteners. Here's Marion Nestle on the matter: "[F]ood chemists process fruit juice until it is basically fruit-flavored sugar, and then reconstitute it. *Fruit concentrate* . . . is a euphemism for sugars."[17]

These six should be taken with a grain of . . . well, sugar. They should be an occasional treat, not a cup-a-day habit. Who doesn't want a slice of birthday cake on their special day? Who doesn't want a bowl of peach ice cream on July Fourth? Who doesn't want an occasional tart from a French bakery? None can be made without refined sugar (or a refined sugar product). But they're treats, not staples.

ALMOST REAL SWEETENERS

The other day, Bruce and I were in Guido's, a high-end market in Great Barrington, Massachusetts. We're always searching the shelves for what's new. Bruce came across unrefined, unbleached, organic whole-cane sugar—sometimes called demerara sugar.

I won't lie: the price almost stopped me dead. It was just under six bucks for a pound and a half—as opposed to four bucks for a 5-pound bag of refined sugar.

But it has revolutionized his baking. It's made from crystallized sugarcane juice; the flavor is pronounced, almost earthy. Pretty close to the real thing, in our opinions. And usable in almost all recipes.

But expensive. Which isn't the worst thing. It means he doesn't pull it out of the pantry all that often. It's not an everyday thing — it's a wonderful new find, used like refined sugar but with way more taste: a little minerally, deep, complex, sophisticated, and intriguing.

There are others in this category:

- turbinado sugar (another raw sugar like demerara but with less molasses left in the batch),
- muscovado sugar (a raw sugar with *more* molasses left in the batch),
- pure cane syrup,
- agave nectar, and even
- maple sugar, made from drying maple syrup and grinding it into grains.

In all cases, the processing is more minimal and the flavors are more intense. In fact, the more we pull back from the factorization of what's sweet, the more flavors we find. Think about wine or beer. Both are sweet but in complex ways, full of notes and flavors: vanilla, citrus, nutty, earthy, tannic, bracing, bright. There are dozens of ways to be sweet. Highly refined products make it seem otherwise.

Lately, there's been a lot of talk about *cane syrup*, the syrup pressed from the sugarcane. It may or may not be refined in various ways. As an overreaction to high-fructose corn syrup, it's sometimes even offered as a moniker for health. *Oh, well, it's got pure cane syrup in it. How bad can it be?* Bad or not, it's still a high-calorie, low-nutrition food.

Therefore, it's like almost all sweeteners in this category. They ring in at 120 calories per ounce and are of little nutritional value.[18] They taste great, but they're not necessary for life.

Want to know how much of those sugars you're eating? Look at the ingredient list on a package; check out the number of grams of sugar per serving. Now divide that number by four. That's the number of teaspoons of sugar you're getting in each serving. (And notice how many servings the package says it contains. It may surprise you.)

Always be cautious of health claims. A candy bar with omega-3 fatty acids is still a candy bar. Do some exploring and discover ways to bake and cook with less-refined sugars. Sweet is a powerful tool, one capable of bringing better satisfaction to dishes. But it should be used wisely and sparingly.

PULLED VEGETABLE SANDWICHES

A sweet touch in a dish not only brightens the flavors, it also adds notes and overtones for flare. The idea for this dish came from barbecue pulled pork sandwiches. In those, the meat is cooked until it can be pulled into threads. Here, the vegetables are shredded, then mixed into a vinegary barbecue sauce to become a terrific filling for buns or toasted bread slices. Serve with pickles, tomatoes, or lettuce—and maybe some Dijon mustard.

1 cup hot, medium, or mild salsa

1 cup unsweetened apple juice, plus more if necessary

¼ cup apple cider vinegar

¼ cup honey

2 tablespoons mild paprika

1 tablespoon dry mustard

1 teaspoon ground allspice

½ teaspoon freshly ground black pepper

2 small yellow-fleshed potatoes (about ¼ pound each), such as a Yukon Golds, shredded through the large holes of a box grater

2 medium carrots, shredded through the large holes of a box grater

1 large Savoy cabbage (about 18 ounces), outer leaves removed, halved, cored, and the remaining leaves shredded through the large holes of a box grater (or 18 ounces bagged, preshredded cabbage)

½ teaspoon kosher salt or fine-grain sea salt

4 whole wheat buns or kaiser rolls

1. Stir the salsa, ½ cup of the apple juice, the vinegar, honey, paprika, dry mustard, allspice, and pepper in a large saucepan set over medium heat.

2. Bring the mixture to a simmer, stir in the potatoes and carrots, and continue simmering for 5 minutes, stirring often.

3. Lay the cabbage on top of the simmering sauce and sprinkle the remaining ½ cup apple juice over it. Do not stir. Cover the pan, reduce the heat to very low, and steam the cabbage for 3 minutes.

4. Stir to thoroughly incorporate the cabbage, cover the pan, and continue cooking until the vegetables are tender and the sauce is quite thick, about 15 minutes, stirring occasionally. If the mixture starts to stick, reduce the heat even further, to the barest flame, then add water in 2 tablespoon increments, until the sauce is thick but not pastelike. If the mixture is too wet and soupy, uncover the pan and raise the heat a bit to let the excess moisture boil away.

5. When the vegetables are tender, remove the pan from the heat, season with salt, and let stand, covered, for 5 minutes. Serve on the buns or rolls.

MAKES 4 SANDWICHES

~~~~~~~

REAL SWEETENERS

1. Honey
In the United States alone, there are more than three hundred recognized varietals, everything from blueberry to acacia, alfalfa to eucalyptus, star thistle to buckwheat. The more flavor, the more intriguing. Here's a basic guide:

FLAVOR	TYPES	USE . . .
Light	Clover, sage and most herbs, alfalfa	As a substitute for sugar in baking; as a drizzle over cheese (particularly feta or blue cheese)

FLAVOR	TYPES	USE ...
Medium	Berry (blueberry, blackberry, raspberry, etc.), orange blossom, star thistle, dandelion, wildflower	On toast or pancakes; in smoothies
Dark	Buckwheat, eucalyptus, oak, pine (and most tree honeys), avocado, certain blends	As a drizzle on roasted root vegetables; in sauces and marinades; as a glaze for roasted meats

Honey requires far fewer steps to get it from the plants (or the hives) to our tables, than, say, refined white sugar from beets. The bees collect nectar, store it in sacs on their bodies, bring it back to the hive, deposit it, thicken it by beating their wings over it, and seal it up with a wax secreted from their glands. The honey is then extracted from the comb, usually by some sort of centripetal machine, and bottled on the spot.

It takes so much nectar to make honey that one bee will produce only about one thimbleful in her lifetime. We certainly reap the benefits!

To inhibit crystallization because of naturally occurring yeasts, some honey is also pasteurized (that is, heated in some way). Proper pasteurization in no way destroys the goodness of honey. However, local producers may sell so-called raw honey, meaning it hasn't been heated in any way. Still and nonetheless, all honey without prior treating will crystallize soon after harvest. Even heated honeys may do so over time.

To prevent crystallization, store honey in a dry, dark place, never in the fridge. If it does crystallize, place the opened bottle in a saucepan of very warm water for five minutes or so. Repeat as necessary until the honey returns to its liquid state.

If you want to substitute honey for sugar in baking, follow these three steps:

1. Use ⅞ cup honey (that is, ¾ cup plus 2 tablespoons) for every cup of sugar.

2. Reduce the liquid in the recipe by 3 tablespoons.

3. Drop the oven temperature by 25°F to prevent over-browning.

Or try this great quick bread, made with honey as well as flavorful walnut oil:

HONEY BANANA BREAD

Here's a great dessert or occasional snack. The bread freezes very well, so cut it into eight slices, wrap each individually in plastic wrap and freeze them—little treats you can take to work over the next few weeks, or pack as snacks for the kids in their lunch boxes. (They'll defrost during the day and be ready by midafternoon.)

¼ cup walnut oil

2 large eggs, at room temperature

¾ cup honey

1 tablespoon vanilla extract

3 large ripe bananas, peeled and the
    flesh mashed a bit with a fork in a
    small bowl

1 cup unbleached all-purpose flour

1 cup whole wheat flour

3 tablespoons toasted wheat germ
    (see Note)

½ teaspoon ground cinnamon

½ teaspoon baking soda

¼ teaspoon fine-grain sea salt

1. Position a rack in the center of the oven and preheat to 325°F. Dab a little walnut oil on a wadded-up paper towel and grease the inside of a 9 x 5-inch loaf pan, taking care to get the oil into the corners and seams.

2. Beat the eggs, honey, walnut oil, and vanilla in a large bowl with an electric mixer at medium speed until creamy, about 2 minutes.

3. Beat in the mashed bananas. Scrape off and remove the beaters.

4. Scrape down the sides of the bowl with a rubber spatula and stir in both flours, the wheat germ, cinnamon, soda, and salt just until any streaks of white flour have disappeared into the moist batter. Pour into the prepared loaf pan.

5. Bake until a toothpick inserted into the center of the bread comes out clean, about 1 hour. Cool in the pan for 5 minutes, then turn out onto a wire rack and continue cooling to room temperature. Cut the loaf into 8 slices to serve.

Note: Wheat germ, the germ (see page 210), from wheat seeds, is sold toasted and untoasted. Toasted offers a deeper, richer taste, a boon for us. Once opened, store it in the refrigerator.

MAKES 8 SERVINGS

~~~~~~

2. Maple Syrup

Although maple syrup may call up images of autumn in New England, the trees are actually tapped while the ground's still deep in snow. We always make a trek out to a farm near us to watch the guys boil down the sap. It descends in the lines from the trees to a big tank in their woodshed.

It's an astounding amount of work. Early in the season, it takes about 20 gallons of sap to make a gallon of syrup; as the season goes on and the sap gets diluted (more groundwater, spring rains), it can take 50, even 70 gallons of sap to make a gallon of syrup.

The flavors develop based on the soil composition and snow amounts over the winter. Up in Vermont and Canada, many people prize the light, delicate syrups that come from hard cold snaps and poor soil. Down in southern New England, the leaf-rot-rich soils produce darker, earthier syrups.

Maple syrup is sold by grades, marked on the bottle. In Vermont, the largest U.S. producer, it's divided into five basic grades: Grade A fancy light amber, Grade A medium amber, Grade A dark amber, Grade B (only for baking), and Grade C (almost like molasses and sold to commercial manufacturers).

Although light amber is the most expensive, Bruce and I prefer medium or even dark amber, slightly stronger and more herbaceous.

Canadian syrup—85 percent of the global supply—is graded like Vermont's with Grade 1 divided into three subsets, followed by Grades 2 and 3. Most other U.S. states grade with fewer categories, but those marked Grade A or AA are always preferred.

If you want to substitute maple syrup for sugar in baking, follow this rule:

Use ¾ cup for every cup of sugar, but also decrease the total amount of liquid in the recipe by about 3 tablespoons for each cup of syrup used.

Or try this delicious recipe, a little bit of New England goodness wherever you are:

WALNUT-DATE SCONES

This breakfast will set you up right on the weekend—assuming you've got some all-fruit spread to go on the side! Squirrel the remaining scones in a sealed plastic bag in the freezer for a breakfast any morning of the week; just leave one on the counter while you shower and get ready, then microwave it for less than a minute to knock off the chill. One more thing: don't be afraid of the buttermilk in this recipe. These days, it's just cultured milk, sort of like a very sour, runny yogurt. It just sounds like it's more fattening than it is.

1 cup unbleached all-purpose flour	½ cup chopped pitted dates
¾ cup whole wheat flour	½ cup regular or low-fat buttermilk
2 teaspoons baking powder	¼ cup toasted walnut oil
¼ teaspoon ground cinnamon	¼ cup maple syrup
¼ teaspoon fine-grain sea salt	½ tablespoon vanilla extract
½ cup walnut pieces, coarsely chopped	

1. Position a rack in the center of the oven and preheat to 375°F. Line a large baking sheet with a silicone baking mat or with parchment paper.

2. Whisk both flours, the baking powder, cinnamon, and salt in a large bowl. Stir in the chopped walnuts and dates.

3. Use a wooden spoon to stir in the buttermilk, walnut oil, maple syrup, and vanilla extract. Keep stirring until fairly smooth, a sort of soft dough, with no white streaks of dry flour visible. However, don't stir too much—just until all the dry ingredients are moistened.

4. Turn the dough out onto a clean, dry work surface and pat it into an 8-inch round that is about ½ inch thick. Use a flatware knife to cut this round into six pie wedges.

5. Divide the wedges and place them on the prepared baking sheet, spacing them a couple inches apart. Bake until browned and toasty on the outside, 15 to 18 minutes. Cool on the tray for 5 minutes before transferring to a wire rack and continuing to cool until you can't wait anymore.

MAKES 6 SCONES

〜〜〜

Putting It All Together: The Real Food Chart

At long last, we can fill in the real food chart for our culinary enhancements:

REAL FOOD	ALMOST REAL FOOD	BARELY REAL FOOD	NOT REAL FOOD
Sea salt, unrefined sea salt, soy sauce, and fish sauce (the last two depending on their components)	Less refined table salt, kosher salt, baking soda	Baking powder, common table salt	MSG, sodium alginate, disodium phosphate, sodium nitrate/nitrite

Cold-pressed olive oil, peanut oil, nut oils, seed oils, butter, lard, schmaltz, duck fat, etc.	Whipped butter (made by whipping nitrogen into butter to make it spreadable—however, some brands include hydrogenated or processed oils. Read those labels!)	Refined oils of any kind, as well as tasteless oils that add nothing except calories and a little lubricant in a saucepan	Hydrogenated oils or fats with additional trans fats
Honey, maple syrup	Raw and unrefined sugars, pure cane syrup, agave nectar, maple sugar, natural molasses	Refined white sugar, standard brown sugar, corn syrup, rice syrup, fruit syrups and concentrates, molasses	Chemical sweeteners, high-fructose corn syrup

PUTTING IT INTO ACTION: A REAL BURGER

Yes, all along we've been hard on burgers. So it's time to enjoy a real one: lean ground meat, tasty buns, and lots of veggies—made even better with a good grasp of how real enhancements bring real satisfaction to a meal.

For each burger, begin with 5 ounces of 95 percent lean ground beef, then add ¼ teaspoon Worcestershire sauce and ¼ teaspoon freshly ground black pepper for each burger. Work the mixture into a patty (or several equal patties if you're making several burgers). Make an indentation with your thumb in the center of the patty to keep it from balling up over the heat.

Heat a skillet over medium heat or fire up the grill. Place the patty in the skillet or on the grill directly over the heat and cook until nicely browned, about 4 minutes. Turn and, if desired, lay one ½-ounce of sliced Brie, Asiago, Gruyère, or Cheddar over the patty. Continue cooking until almost cooked through, maybe about 3 minutes (or to be more accurate, until an instant-read meat thermometer inserted into the center of the patty registers about 140°F).

Remove the patty from the heat; set it on a whole wheat bun with a couple Romaine lettuce leaves and a couple Roma tomato slices.

At only 430 calories (with the Brie) and less salt, fat, and sugars than a chain-restaurant version, this is real food: satisfying, simple, and unshellacked. That's what Bruce and I were craving that day at lunch near the mall. That's what we've all been craving.

REAL TOPPINGS

Want more flavor? Here are toppings for a single burger. You can increase their volume at will, adding more veggies to every bite.

✦ For a sautéed zucchini topping, shred a medium zucchini through the large holes of a box grater. Add about a teaspoon of olive oil to a large skillet, set it over medium-high heat, and add the zucchini. Toss and stir just until barely wilted, about 3 minutes. Then add a little finely grated lemon zest.

✦ Sauté 1 cup sliced mushrooms in a skillet over medium heat with 1 teaspoon olive oil, avocado oil, or unsalted butter. Stir until the mushrooms give up their liquid and it evaporates to a thick glaze, about 5 minutes. You're looking for an increase of moisture in the skillet, then that liquid to bubble down to almost nothing. Season with a few dashes of hot red pepper sauce, such as Tabasco sauce.

✦ Set a red bell pepper or a spicy poblano chile directly over the heat on the grill or 4 inches from a preheated broiler on a baking sheet. Don't poke, slice, or cut the pepper or chile in any way. Grill or broil, turning occasionally, until blackened on all sides. Then place in a small bowl and cover with plastic wrap. Set aside for 10 minutes. Peel off most of the blackened stuff, then cut off the stem and slice the pepper or chile into strips, getting rid of the seeds and any white membranes inside. Try not to put the pepper or chile under running water to get the blackened bits off, despite their turning sticky. Rinse your hands, then go back to work.

✦ For a peppery bite, shred a couple radishes through the large holes of a box grater, then toss them with a spritz of lime juice and a pinch of ground cumin.

✦ Make a salad burger by dressing 1 cup arugula with 2 teaspoons balsamic vinegar and 1 teaspoon olive oil. Pile this on top of the burger and eat it with a fork.

✦ Put a carrot slaw on top of the burger. Shred a carrot through the large holes of a box grater, then toss with a couple teaspoons of rice vinegar (and even some sesame seeds if you want to get fancy)—yet another pile-up of real food.

✦ Don't forget a nest of radish or vegetable sprouts on a burger, a summery treat.

REAL CONDIMENTS

Don't stop at toppings. Burgers need condiments. Forget those laced with high-fructose corn syrup or chemical fake-outs. Here are some that will set your meal dancing:

✦ Chinese chile paste

✦ Jamaican Pickapeppa Sauce

✦ Sambal (an Indonesian hot sauce)

✦ Pomegranate molasses, a thickened Middle Eastern sweet/sour sauce

✦ For your own deli mustard, put ¾ cup yellow mustard seeds, 1½ teaspoons kosher salt, 1½ teaspoons freshly ground black pepper, ¼ teaspoon ground cinnamon, ¼ teaspoon ground allspice, ⅛ teaspoon ground cloves, and ⅛ teaspoon ground mace in a large bowl. Stir in ¾ cup dark beer and ½ cup white wine vinegar. Cover and set aside at room temperature for 2 days. Pour the whole thing into a large blender or a food processor, then blend or process for about 4 minutes, stopping the machine every once in a while and scraping down the inside walls of the canister. You'll think nothing's happening at first, then the mustard seeds will begin to break down and the whole thing will start to thicken. Keep blending or processing until it's coarse-grained deli mustard. Scrape the contents into a bowl, cover, and refrigerate overnight before using—then store, covered, in the refrigerator for up to 4 months.

✦ A tablespoon of pecan pesto can really do the trick. First toast ¼ cup pecan halves in a dry skillet over medium-low heat until aromatic and lightly browned, stirring occasionally, about 3 minutes. You'll also hear them sizzle when the fat inside the nuts starts to get charged up. Pour these into a large food processor fitted with the chopping blade, then add 2 cups packed basil leaves, 3 tablespoons olive oil, 3 tablespoons water, a couple slivered garlic cloves, a few grinds of black pepper, and 1½ ounces finely grated Parmigiano-Reggiano; grind until it becomes a coarse paste, scraping down the insides of the canister once or twice to make sure everything takes a spin on the blades. Scrape the pesto into a bowl and serve at once or store in the fridge for up to 1 week (to keep it from going brown, press plastic wrap right on top of the pesto after it's been in the chill for about 1 hour).

STEP

5

Take the Long View

WHAT WILL YOU DO?

Begin to say "Yes, and . . ." to real food

Explore your supermarket's produce section

Build a better pantry

Keep a one- or two-day journal

～～～～～～～～～～

WHAT WILL YOU DISCOVER?

How to be open to possibilities

Tips for shopping and discovering even more
real food, including international foods

How to take stock and evaluate it

The *Yes, And* Life

It started out as small irritations during cooking demonstrations.

"Let me show you how to stem that thyme."

"Aren't you done chopping that onion yet?"

Then it grew into a low-grade war. All because Bruce was afraid I was going to screw up on camera and I was insecure enough to think he was going to show me up.

On NBC's *Today* show, I actually heard myself say, "He's showing you the cheffy way to do it. I'll show you the real way."

Mind you, Bruce *is* a trained chef. He knows *the real way*. I, the writer, have a more homey technique.

Our insecurities were getting in the way, as they always do. They stop growth. Flow too. Even fun. Who can take the long view, head down in fear?

We decided to fix the problem. I went into therapy and Bruce enrolled in improvisational comedy classes. (We all have our ways of coping.)

Improv taught him to stay fluid, accepting what came at him while making something out of it. One of the games he learned was called *Yes, And*. As he built a scene, no matter what anyone said, he had to answer with "Yes, and . . ." Like this:

Person 1: "I believe politicians are honest."

Person 2: "Yes, and I've always wondered what planet you live on."

Person 1: "Yes, Jupiter. And my whole family is in politics."

It didn't take us long to figure out that *Yes, And* was the perfect attitude toward food. Presented with something new, many of us back up. Or even walk away—only to fall into ruts. Like the same dinner every night, the same snack every afternoon: this take-out, that candy bar. That's mostly fear—of change, of difference, of alternatives, of effort. In any case, it's a sure way to remain closed to pleasure.

Detoxed Palates Can Change

We're born with few proclivities besides a drive for the sweet stuff found in our mothers' milk.[1] We don't come into the world disliking spinach. We learn to. Believe it or not. Our mothers are afraid we won't like it, we read the reaction in their faces, and we back up, suddenly fearful.

But that's actually the good news. We learn—and can grow. Not long after our *Yes, And* commitment to food, I watched a real change happen with Bruce. When I met him, he didn't eat anything that lived in water. Me? I love seafood: fried fish, lobster salad—but mostly sushi. At Japanese restaurants in New York, I'd order my favorites while Bruce chomped the chicken yakitori, carefully studying my reactions. (Think of *When Harry Met Sally.*)

One evening, he asked if I'd order him one piece of tuna. "But on your plate, not mine," he said.

I was shocked but quickly complied.

He didn't wolf it down, a childish urge to get it out of his mouth. Instead, he slowed down, really trying to savor it. He was clearly shocked at the velvety creaminess.

The next time, he asked me to order him two pieces of tuna.

Then one day, I watched him order sea urchin on his own.

"Did you know you officially like seafood?" I asked.

He nodded and took another bite.

We adults are neither a blank slate nor a filled-up canvas. We have pleasurable memories of the foods we love *and* the ability to lay down new tracks. What we didn't like as kids, we might well like now, particularly once we detox from the excessive salt-fat-sugar shellac *and* if we follow our basic tasting guidelines: finding flavor overtones, chewing well, relishing a range of textures, and imagining other foods similar to the one we are eating.

When faced with a new food, do what Bruce did: prime yourself for a *Yes, And* reaction. First, take a deep breath and relax your jaw so there's no tension. Take a bite, put your hands down, and open your mind. (If you really want to go all out, open your hands, too.) Close your eyes. And breathe deeply. You're on your way to laying down new memory tracks by accepting bits and pieces of the full world of real food: fruits, berries, vegetables, herbs, seeds, grains, nuts, fungi, fish, mollusks, bivalves, shellfish, pigs, cows, rabbits, birds, sugars, and fats.

We have a friend who always turned up her nose at leafy greens. Once when she spent the weekend with us, Bruce was testing pizza recipes for a new book. One of the pies included Swiss chard, cherry tomatoes, and blue cheese. The flavors were complex, but the greens offered a bit of savory earthiness under the acid pop of the tomatoes and the creamy cheese. Our friend looked askance at the slice. "Okay, I'll trust you," she said before she took a bite.

We could both see the reaction. "Hey," she mumbled, her mouth full, "I think I like Swiss chard."

And probably more greens, too. Because with real food's flavor overtones and textural range, everything leads to something else. If you like coffee, soon enough you'll like red wine or mushrooms or Chinese black bean sauce, all because you find a common, mellow earthiness among them. If you like vanilla, you may well like cantaloupe, celery root, and buttercup squash. After Bruce learned to like sushi, he also lost his aversion to mayonnaise, probably because of flavor and textural resonances.

Still, many of us lead with fear and are severely limited when it comes to what we eat because of:

✦ entrenched habits

✦ what we find on the supermarket shelves

✦ and the overgrowth of a food media in which chefs cook the same meal over and over again: a big sweating hunk of protein, a puny side vegetables, and a gorgeous dessert

Admittedly, we can't do much about the third problem, other than to acknowledge it. But we can change the first two. We'll save the second one for later in this step. Let's take on the first, entrenched habits, right now. We'll start with a few small changes. We'll take three favorite dishes and tweak them slightly to make them even more enjoyable, opening our palates to new tastes.

GRILLED CAESAR SALAD

Remember the first time you had a chicken breast off a grill, rather than out of a skillet? The new taste was probably a revelation. Here, we're going to alter a classic salad with a similar twist. The lettuces are grilled to add a little char and a slightly sweeter mellowness. One little shift and your perspective changes, your enjoyment deepens. To make this a main-course entrée, add some purchased, cooked cocktail shrimp or the skinned and boned meat off a rotisseried chicken from the supermarket.

2 large Romaine lettuce heads

1 small radicchio head

3 tablespoons olive oil

3 tablespoons balsamic vinegar

1 teaspoon Dijon mustard

1 garlic clove, pressed through a
   garlic press or very finely minced

½ teaspoon freshly ground black
   pepper

¼ teaspoon fine-grain sea salt

1 ounce Parmigiano-Reggiano,
   shaved into thin strips with a
   vegetable peeler

1. Prepare a grill for high-heat cooking or heat a grill pan over medium-high heat.

2. Cut both Romaine heads and the radicchio head in half through the root ends. Rinse out the inner leaves to remove any grit, then shake them dry over the sink.

3. Drizzle the oil over the cut sides of the lettuces, then set them cut side down on the grate directly over the heat on a grill or on a grill pan. Grill until lightly browned and a little wilted, about 5 minutes. Do not turn.

4. Transfer to a cutting board and chop into bite-size bits, removing the tough core at the root end. Place the lettuce shreds in a large serving bowl.

5. Whisk the vinegar, mustard, garlic, pepper, and salt in a small bowl. Pour over the lettuce, add the cheese, and toss well.

MAKES 4 SERVINGS

CHICKEN BREASTS SAUTÉED WITH RADISHES

Another way to practice *Yes, And* is to add a new ingredient to an old favorite. In this weeknight recipe, Bruce has added a surprise: radishes. When cooked, they turn sweet, creamy, and sophisticated.

2 tablespoons olive oil

Four 5-ounce boneless, skinless chicken breasts (see Note)

½ teaspoon freshly ground black pepper

8 large radishes, thinly sliced

½ cup rosé wine, dry vermouth, or reduced-sodium fat-free chicken broth

1 tablespoon white wine vinegar

1 tablespoon unsalted butter

¼ teaspoon kosher salt or fine-grain sea salt

1. Heat a large skillet over medium heat. Swirl in the oil. Slip the chicken breasts into the skillet. Sprinkle them with half the pepper, then cook until well browned, 5 or 6 minutes.

2. Turn the breasts, sprinkle with the remaining pepper, and continue cooking until well browned on the other side, until an instant-read meat thermometer inserted into the thickest part of one breast registers 165°F, about 5 more minutes. Transfer to four serving plates.

3. Add the radishes to the skillet. Cook, stirring often, for 2 minutes.

4. Pour in the wine or its substitutes; bring to a simmer, scraping up any browned bits on the skillet's bottom. Continue cooking until the wine has reduced to about half its original volume, about 1 minute.

5. Whisk in the vinegar and butter until the butter melts and thickens the sauce a bit. Whisk in the salt and divide the sauce among the breasts.

Note: There's one trick to making sure chicken breasts are never overcooked—but it does take a bit more time. Mix ¼ cup kosher salt with 8 cups cool water in a large bowl, then submerge the breasts in the solution. Refrigerate for 2 to 4 hours, then remove the breasts from the brine and rinse before using. If you use this tip, omit the salt from this (or any) recipe.

MAKES 4 SERVINGS

CLOCKWISE: **Fresh Peach Salsa;
Thyme and Garlic-Roasted Shrimp;
Spaghetti with Sausage, Carrots,
and Frisée; Salmon with Salsa**

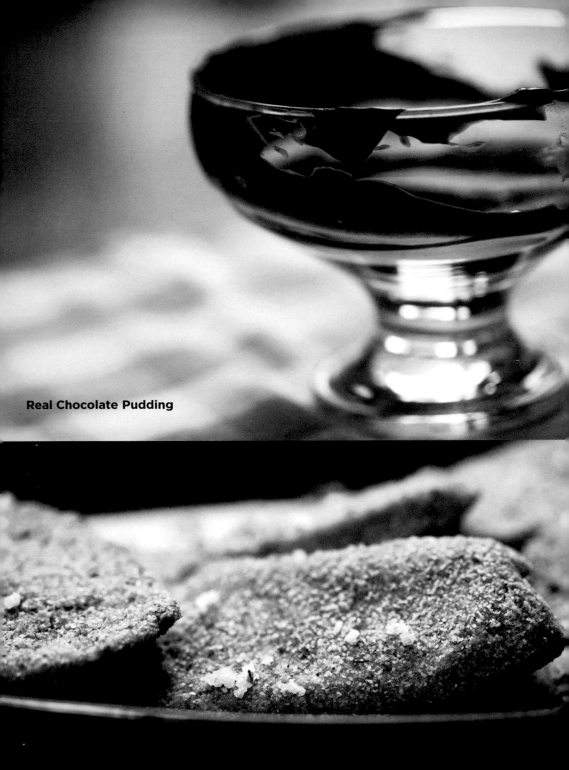

Real Chocolate Pudding

Oven-Fried Fish Fillets

Zucchini Cakes

Skillet Macaroni and Broccoli and Mushrooms and Cheese

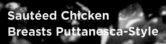

**Sautéed Chicken
Breasts Puttanesca-Style**

Fish Fillets in Packets

Mapo Dofu

A Real Burger with
Carrot Slaw and Sambal

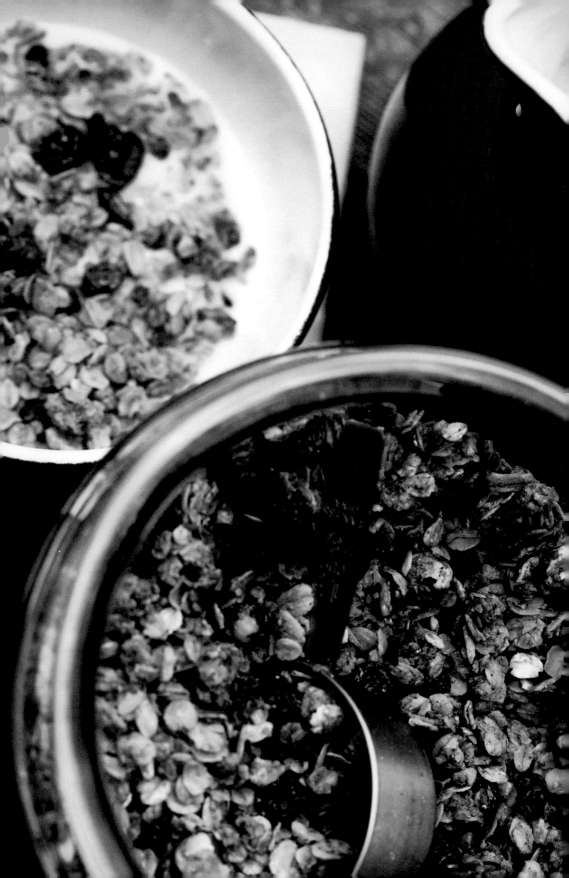

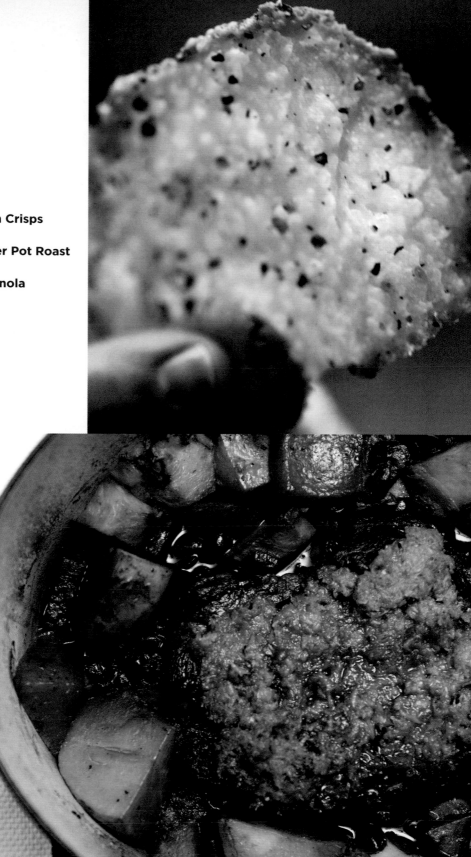

RIGHT: **Parmesan Crisps**

BELOW: **Best-Ever Pot Roast**

FACING PAGE: **Granola**

TOP: **Panzanella**

BOTTOM: **Raspberry Crisp;
Chocolate-Chunk Oatmeal Cookies**

FETTUCCINI WITH MUSHROOMS

Another way to open up to new possibilities is to explore the variety of a single ingredient—like mushrooms. By mixing rarer varieties with more economical ones, you'll experience new flavors in an old favorite.

1 tablespoon olive oil

1 tablespoon unsalted butter

3 medium shallots, minced

8 ounces cremini or brown button mushrooms, thinly sliced

6 ounces portobello caps, thinly sliced

3½ ounces shiitake mushrooms, the stems removed and discarded, the caps thinly sliced

2 teaspoons stemmed thyme leaves or 1 teaspoon dried thyme

½ teaspoon red pepper flakes

2 medium garlic cloves, minced

⅔ cup dry white wine, dry vermouth, or reduced-sodium vegetable broth

9 ounces fresh fettuccini, cooked and drained according to the package's instructions

2 ounces Parmigiano-Reggiano, finely grated

¼ teaspoon fine-grain sea salt

1. Heat a large skillet over medium heat. Add the oil and butter; tilt the skillet over the heat until the butter melts.

2. Toss in the shallots. Cook, stirring often, until softened, about 2 minutes.

3. Pour in all three types of mushrooms. Cook, stirring occasionally, until they give off their liquid and it evaporates to a glaze, about 7 minutes.

4. Add the thyme, red pepper flakes, and garlic; stir over the heat until very aromatic, about 15 seconds. Then pour in the wine, vermouth, or broth. Bring to a simmer, scraping up any browned bits on the skillet's bottom.

5. Continue simmering until the wine, or its substitutes, has reduced to about two-thirds of its original volume, maybe 1 or 2 minutes.

6. Plop the cooked pasta into the skillet. Add the cheese and salt. Remove from the heat and toss well until the pasta is thoroughly mixed into the mushrooms.

MAKES 4 SERVINGS

One New Thing

Years ago, I lived in Austin, Texas, a few blocks from a grocery store billed as a gourmet's heaven: aisles of small-batch products and a sign that once read *Forty-seven varieties of apples!*

Forty-seven? I was undone. And not much of an apple eater. I mean, I grew up down south, hundreds of miles from most apple orchards.

That day, I bought one each of many varietals: prairie spy, northern spy, Cox's orange pippin, golden pippin, Bramley's seedling, and Brownlee's russet. By the next day, I was a committed apple eater because I had practiced a *Yes, And* life and had gone out of my way to find more possibilities, exploring a supermarket with a wider range.

Make this your goal, too. Spend a few minutes this week finding a supermarket with a better produce section—perhaps through an Internet search or by a friend's recommendation. Will it take an extra fifteen minutes to get there? Maybe. But you'll find more to explore—and therefore to enjoy. It need not be an expensive, gourmet supermarket; you simply want one that foregrounds a big selection of fresh fruits and vegetables, maybe even with a commitment to local growers.

Take a spin around the produce section and see what's there. An apple or pear you've never heard of? Pick it up, look at it, smell it, study it.

Walk over to the lettuces, probably part of a whole wall. Some are bagged; others, in full heads. How many have you tried? Mâche, radicchio, baby oak leaf? Which ones have a distinct smell? Those will taste bigger, bolder, maybe astringent, maybe sweeter. They'll probably need bolder dressings: creamy, with some cheese in the mix.

Look at the herbs, then check out the citrus. How would you prepare the new things you're finding? How would you find recipes? And how would you enjoy the dishes?

Somewhere nearby, there are bins of aromatics, the foundation of almost all the dishes we cook, all members of the lily family. These are the basic four in any grocery store:

1. Onions. Yellow are mild; red, sweet; and white, assertive. Supersweet onions like Vidalias are of little benefit in cooking and should be eaten raw on burgers or in salads.

2. Shallots. You've already seen them a lot in Bruce's recipes. They're like a cross between garlic and an onion. Many come with two cloves per head (although there are single-clove varieties on the market as well).

3. Leeks. These long, skinny vegetables add an incredible earthiness to many dishes. When cooking, use only the white and pale green parts. Remove the root threads, then slice this bottom section in half lengthwise to carefully wash its inner chambers of sand before slicing it up.

4. Scallions. These have a bright, heady taste, spring in every bite. They're fully edible (with the possible exception of those stringy root threads dangling off the lobe).

One way to practice a *Yes, And* life is to switch out one aromatic for another in any recipe: a sweeter red onion for a more astringent white one; some garlicky shallots for a yellow onion; some mellow leeks instead of shallots; some bright scallions instead of a blander onion. Of course, volumes change; but you can eyeball the difference in any recipe.

Now that you've visited that produce section and explored the possibilities, make this pledge:

✦ I will do my best to try one new fruit, vegetable, meat, fish, food preparation, or recipe every week.

Maybe it's hake, tarragon, or a kumquat. Maybe it's that bottle of blueberry ketchup on the store shelf, a new breed of plum you've never seen before, or simply an ingredient prepared in a new way. Maybe it's a recipe from this book or another cookbook.

Look to the future, anticipating pleasure. What foods do you imagine you'll try in the weeks ahead? Are there things you've always wanted to give a whirl?

Will you be able to try one new thing every week? Maybe not. Sometimes life gets in the way. But the point is the commitment.

In a few short weeks, you'll have a new set of tastes, new memory tracks, an ever-expanding palate, and a life open to change. But don't stop there. Keep finding more. Yes, and . . .

Eat More Things to Eat Less

Here's the real reason to make this *Yes, And* commitment: when we expand our range, we eat less because we're satisfied more quickly. Boredom clearly leads to overeating.[2] And boredom extends to what's on our plates.

Say you eat a big plate of salad greens for lunch, maybe with some tomatoes and cucumbers in the mix, all dressed in a vinaigrette. Chances are, you'll be hungry in a few hours. The variety was dull; the satisfaction, limited.

But if you eat a plate that has a third of that salad, along with some tabbouleh (see pages 47–48) and a heaping spoonful of guacamole, you'll be less hungry all afternoon because you broadened the range with lots of textures and flavors that together overturn boredom and lead to greater satiety. With more food choices, you're satisfied more quickly at the table and you stay sated longer. That's a winning strategy!

Eating the same thing again and again is palliative, about like taking a palate tranquilizer. Sure, I love mac-and-cheese. But there would be little point in eating it once a week. It would soon become a way to soothe fears and calm down not only my taste buds but probably my life, too. That's not the point of food! That's the point of a bath, or a walk, or a favorite movie while snuggled down in the den.

Food must not anesthetize. It has to stimulate. So push the boundaries a bit with recipes like these, full of tastes and flavors you might not have experienced. Choose one or two; make it a goal to experience something beyond the usual repertoire.

SAUTÉED DUCK BREASTS

Here's a supper that looks fancy but really isn't since duck breasts are available in almost every supermarket. Look for plump, firm pieces of meat. Serve them with some mashed potatoes or an easy salad of sliced cucumbers and red onions, tossed with a little rice vinegar and toasted sesame oil.

3 medium duck breasts (about 1½ pounds total weight)

1 tablespoon unsalted butter

2 medium shallots, minced

2 teaspoons honey

2 teaspoons stemmed thyme leaves or 1 teaspoon dried thyme

1 cup dry white wine, dry vermouth, or reduced-sodium vegetable broth

½ teaspoon kosher salt or fine-grain sea salt

½ teaspoon freshly ground black pepper

1. Position a rack in the center of the oven and preheat to 400°F. Use a sharp knife to score lines to make a crosshatch pattern in the creamy, beige fat of the duck breasts, cutting down through the fat but not into the meat.

2. Put the breasts fat side down in a cool, oven-safe skillet; set it over medium heat. Cook for 6 to 8 minutes, until the fat has rendered out and the remaining skin is lusciously crisp.

3. Turn the breasts over and set the skillet in the oven. Roast until an instant-read meat thermometer inserted into one of the breasts registers 140°F for rare or 150°F for medium, about 5 minutes. (The meat should still have a pinkish hue, even when cooked to medium.)

4. Be careful: the skillet's hot. Set it on the stove and transfer the duck breasts to a large cutting board. Drain the fat from the skillet. (Not down the drain, unless you're on very good terms with a plumber. Instead, pour it into a disposable jar, then seal and discard it.)

5. Set the skillet over medium heat and swirl in the butter. Add the shallots and cook, stirring often, until soft, about 2 minutes.

6. Add the honey and thyme. Cook for 30 seconds, then pour in the wine or its substitutes, and bring to a simmer. Continue simmering until it has reduced to half its original volume, about 2 minutes. Stir in the salt and pepper; set aside.

7. Position the breasts on a cutting board so their narrower ends are to your left and right. Slice them into thin bits from one narrow end to the other. Divide these among four serving plates. Spoon the sauce on top.

MAKES 4 SERVINGS

FUYU PERSIMMON SALAD

There are two types of persimmons: the orange fuyu that can be eaten right away and the darker, squishier hachiya, which must be ripened through a hard frost. Make sure you get the fuyus, now common from California and sort of like a squat tomato with a sweet fragrance.

4 cups baby arugula leaves

1½ tablespoons olive oil

3 ripe Fuyu persimmons, stemmed
and sliced into thin wedges

1 very small red onion, sliced into
thin rings

¼ cup toasted walnut pieces, chopped

1½ tablespoons balsamic vinegar

½ teaspoon kosher salt or fine-grain
sea salt

1. Toss the arugula with the oil in a large bowl. Spread onto a serving platter.

2. Top with the sliced persimmons, onion rings, and nuts.

3. Drizzle with the vinegar; sprinkle with salt.

MAKES 4 SERVINGS

ESCAROLE, WHITE BEAN, AND ROASTED GARLIC SOUP

Escarole is a bitter green, prized in Italian cooking because it turns wonderfully sweet over the heat. The heads can be sandy, so make sure you separate the leaves from the root ball to rinse them individually before chopping them. And here's a surprise: this soup includes a poached egg in every bowl. For the best taste, make sure the egg yolks are still a bit runny so they'll melt into the individual servings when broken.

6 garlic cloves, unpeeled (see Note)

1 tablespoon olive oil

3 ounces nitrate-free or uncured pork or beef bacon, finely chopped

1 large yellow onion, finely chopped

1 medium carrot, peeled and thinly sliced

2 medium escarole heads (about 1 pound each), cored, shredded, and washed, but not dried

6 cups fat-free, reduced-sodium chicken broth

1 tablespoon sage leaves, chopped

1 teaspoon finely grated lemon zest (use the small holes of a box grater or a fine-mesh handheld grater)

3½ cups canned cannellini or other small white beans, drained and rinsed

2 teaspoons lemon juice

2 ounces Parmigiano-Reggiano, finely grated

½ teaspoon freshly ground black pepper

4 large eggs

½ teaspoon fine-grain sea salt

1. Preheat the oven to 400°F. Wrap the unpeeled garlic cloves in aluminum foil, then bake until softened and fragrant, about 25 minutes.

2. Heat a large saucepan or soup pot over medium heat. Swirl in the oil, add the bacon, and sauté until browned and sizzling at the edges, stirring frequently, about 2 minutes.

3. Add the onion and carrot. Cook until the onion is pale but fragrant, stirring often, about 2 minutes.

4. Add the escarole and cook just until the greens begin to wilt, tossing constantly, about 2 minutes.

5. Stir in the broth, sage, and lemon zest. Raise the heat to high and bring to a full simmer.

6. Reserve ½ cup of the beans in a small bowl; stir the remainder into the soup. Cover the saucepan, reduce the heat to low, and simmer for 20 minutes.

7. Meanwhile, squeeze the roasted garlic pulp from its hulls into the bowl with the reserved beans. Add the lemon juice and mash with a fork until smooth.

8. After the soup has cooked for 20 minutes, whisk a small amount of the soup broth into the bean puree; stir this combined mixture back into the soup. Stir in the cheese and pepper.

9. Turn off the heat. Crack the eggs one at a time into a small custard cup or other small bowl and slip them into the soup. Cover the pot and let the eggs steep until soft-set, 4 to 5 minutes, depending on how runny you like the yolks.

10. Use a large ladle to gather the eggs up one by one from the soup, placing them in individual serving bowls. You may have to go fishing for them, but do so very gently so as not to break the eggs. Then ladle the soup into the bowls around the eggs. Sprinkle each with a little salt.

Note: Roasted garlic cloves can sometimes be found on your supermarket's salad bar. If desired, buy six of these (so long as they're soft) and skip step 1 entirely.

MAKES 4 SERVINGS

Ever More New Things at Your Local Supermarket

A grocery store is the best place to practice our *Yes, And* life.

However, it *can* feel like a maze: stacks in aisles, bins everywhere, meat that's refrigerated, meat that's not, produce at every turn, fresh, canned, and frozen. I asked Marion Nestle for her take on the matter. "Supermarkets are very large, have lots of products, arrange them in complicated ways, and are not much fun to navigate," she said. "If you've got a routine that gets you out of there in some reasonable amount of time, I can understand why you would want to stick with it. Stores do everything they can to get people to linger, so you are fighting those marketing strategies. This means that every store encounter is a conflict between desire to get what you want and to get out of there."[3]

While taking a *Yes, And* attitude to the supermarket brings greater satisfaction to the table, *getting out* is still the goal. With that in mind, let's lay down two guidelines for our new shopping experiences:

✦ Go in with a plan (a.k.a. a list). This will direct you to real food, helping you avoid the acres of the fake that take up so much real estate.

✦ Don't shop hungry. You're more likely to pick up processed and packaged food, a ready salve for a grumbling stomach. You're also more likely to go off your list, turning an eye to whatever looks good. Instead, go grocery shopping after lunch—or after breakfast on the weekend.

To get in and out while still staying open to at least one new thing a week, here's what to look for:

THE PRODUCE SECTION

We've already taken a spin around this section, but as you go back for more, keep in mind that produce should be fresh, fragrant, and delectable. If it doesn't smell like much, it probably won't taste like much. No amount of snipped herbs and cold-pressed oils will make up for bendy carrots, squishy lettuce, or woody asparagus.

Look beyond gimmicky packaging. On a recent trip, we found premade, packaged guacamole in an over-the-top festive container hanging from a clip in the produce section. We both rolled our eyes—then checked the ingredient list. To our shock, there wasn't a preservative in the batch, not even citric acid. It was real food all the way!

Yes, be on the lookout for sales; but buy only what you will use. A big bag of oranges for a couple bucks is a great deal—but only if you will honestly eat the whole lot before they mold or desiccate into hockey pucks.

And while we're speaking of spoilage, keep in mind that pre-prepped vegetables will not last as long as their whole versions. A container of cubed butternut squash can go soggy in two or three days; whereas a whole butternut squash can last a couple weeks. Still, the payoff of prepared veggies for a busy life cannot be underestimated.

And here's another tip for a busy life: make a trip to the supermarket's or your corner bodega's salad bar when you need small quantities of vegetables. Does a recipe call for some shredded carrots? What about one celery rib? If you don't want to buy the whole bunch, they may well be included in the salad bar. While these cost more per pound, you may also save money by buying a smaller quantity. Fifty cents for those two celery ribs from the salad bar is cheaper than $1.49 for a whole head that will only go boggy in the fridge.

THE DELI

This counter can be a disaster area for real-food mavens. After all, we can't read the ingredient list on that big deli ham without making the clerk haul the thing out and plop it on the counter while we try to see the greasy label on the underside.

How can we make good choices? Keep this guideline in mind:

✦ No part of a turkey, chicken, or pig looks like a football.

Instead, look for the in-store roasted ham, beef, turkey, and chicken: meat shaped like what it is—a roasted turkey breast on a platter, for example. And ask a few questions: How fresh is it? When was it roasted? What's in the marinade?

THE CHEESE CASE

Follow similar advice:

✦ Look for cheese either in cuts and wedges, or sold as full wheels, logs, or pyramids.

What should you avoid?

1. Anything labeled as *cheese food*. Chances are, it's not real food.

2. The spreadable stuff. With the exception of cream cheese, soft goat cheese, and a few other cultured products, no cheese is spreadable without lots of processing. We spotted a package called spreadable feta the other day. Sure enough, it was stocked with gums, acids, and *natural flavors*.

3. Precrumbled cheeses. Many are lathered with cellulose to keep them from clumping and then doped with natamycin, an antifungal agent that may have a negative impact on bacteria necessary for good digestive health. That said, preshredded mozzarella may well be a great time-saver, provided there's nothing chemical in the mix. You know the drill: read the labels. The more informed you are, the better fed you'll be.

THE MEAT CASE

This bewildering variety probably stretches along a whole wall, not to mention a nearby specialty case with prime cuts. It can lure us into a rut, the same-old-same-old.

Fight back! Switch out cuts of meat in favorite recipes, based on the amount of time they need to cook. Sure, there are subtle differences, but if you make a distinction between quick cookers (in five to fifteen minutes) and things that need a longer braise (more than an hour), you can begin to play around with your favorite recipes, tweaking them to find new tastes and experiences.

To make sense of what's there and how long you'll need to cook it, here's a reference chart:

QUICK-COOKING CUTS	LONG-COOKING CUTS
Beef: flank steak, sirloin, strip steaks, rib-eye steaks, T-bone steaks, porterhouse steaks, tenderloin steaks (a.k.a. filet mignon), London broil, liver	Beef: brisket, chuck roast, blade steaks, bottom round, ox tails, eye round, stew meat, shanks, whole tenderloin roast, standing rib roast, tongue
Chicken: boneless, skinless chicken breasts	Chicken: all other cuts
Duck: breasts	Duck: legs, whole birds
Lamb: loin chops, rib chops, loin, sirloin, rack of lamb	Lamb: shoulder chops, legs, stew meat, breasts, shanks
Pork: loin chops, rib chops, tenderloin, bacon, boneless center-cut chops	Pork: whole pork loin, ham, shanks, shoulder, Boston butt, belly, rib roasts
Turkey: scaloppine, turkey London broil	Turkey: whole breasts, leg quarters, wings, whole birds
Veal: scaloppini, rib chops, loin chops (a.k.a. veal porterhouse steaks or veal T-bone steaks)	Veal: brisket, legs, breasts, rib roast, stew meat

Beyond that, remember that a package of beef should include only beef; chicken, chicken; pork, pork. Steer clear of fillers, additives, flavorings, and other industrial mishmash. Also, forget premarinated or prestuffed entrées, mostly doped with corn syrup, preservatives, and even artificial flavors. Instead, look for high-quality, straightforward meats. Do any marinating and stuffing at home.

Don't be afraid to talk to the butchers. Ask what they like. Ask what's fresh, on sale, a good value. If you're in doubt, ask for a package to be opened in front of you. You'll be able to tell if the meat is fresh at the first whiff.

Finally, skip the preground meats in the case. Instead, pick out a sirloin, turkey breast, or boneless country-style pork ribs and ask the butcher to grind them for you. Better ground beef makes for better meals.

THE FISH COUNTER

You can judge a supermarket by its fish counter. If the fillets look mushy, if the shrimp is flattened, and if the scallops are sitting in a milky backwash, go elsewhere.

Other than that, keep in mind that fresh fish should smell fresh. Don't buy packaged, thawed fish, sealed under plastic wrap. How can you tell if it's fresh? If you must, have someone open the package so you can take a whiff.

But also check out the fillets, scallops, and shrimp in the freezer case. Although that array on the counter's ice may look fantastic, most of it was flash-frozen at catch. The shrimp has most likely been defrosted in the back. Better then to go buy the big bag of frozen shrimp and thaw it yourself, saving money all the while. There's little reason to buy the already thawed stuff unless there's a direct claim to its being *never frozen* or it's 6:00 p.m. and you have no time to let something defrost before dinner. In this case, pay for convenience, not aesthetics.[4]

THE DAIRY DEPARTMENT

Is anything better than whole milk or yogurt? Besides the taste factor, there's even a nutritional benefit to the full-fat stuff. Certain vitamins like A and D are fat soluble.

Full-fat dairy is so rich and pleasurable, it can bring satiety faster—if you slow down to feel the cues. However, dairy is often treated as food on the run: milk on cereal as you're trying to get out the door in the morning or yogurt as a snack at your desk midafternoon. Even cheese can be an afterthought with little added taste, the way it was on our burgers by the mall.

There's no doubt: dairy is real food. But for heart health and weight control, it may well be best to choose low-fat dairy offerings. Read those labels! Better to have more fat than a bunch of chemicals and a metallic tang on the tongue.

However, there are two, thick, fat-free yogurts that hit the spot:

✦ Greek-style yogurt, prestrained of its whey to be thick and luscious

✦ Skyr, an Icelandic fat-free yogurt cultured until it's rich and decadent, sort of like very soft cream cheese

THE CENTRAL AISLES

A supermarket is an apartment building; every producer rents shelf space. The guy who pays the most gets the prime position at eye level.

Are many of these products real food? Of course. But don't miss what's in less-prime real estate. The turbinado sugar is often on the bottom shelf; the nut oils, up top. To try one new thing a week, you have to look up and down.

You'll also find an amazing number of international products. Back in the day (and we're talking the mid-eighties), olive oil was exotic, hard to find in neighborhood supermarkets. Nowadays, almost all supermarkets have one if not several international aisles, stocked with the basics from around the world. This is good news for real-food lovers! You can expand your palate, press the boundaries further, and create new food experiences right from your neighborhood grocery store.

But remember the real-food rules: read those labels on international products to make sure that, say, the Chinese bean sauce you're buying has no chemical preservatives or fake-out shenanigans. Then say, "Yes, and . . ." to the wider world of food by whipping up some international favorites right from your local supermarket. Here are six recipes to get you started:

DUKKAH

This Egyptian spice-and-nut blend can be used as a dip for whole wheat pita bread or celery sticks. It's a great condiment to serve on the side of a plate of salads and vegetables, a way to add more flavors and thus more pleasure to the meal.

½ cup walnuts, pecans, or hazelnuts

¼ cup whole coriander seeds

2 tablespoons white or black sesame seeds

2 tablespoons whole cumin seeds

1 tablespoon whole black peppercorns

1 teaspoon fennel seeds

¼ cup walnut, pecan, or hazelnut oil (to match the nuts you've chosen)

1 teaspoon kosher salt or fine-grain sea salt

1. Preheat the oven to 325°F. Spread the nuts on a large, lipped baking sheet, then set them in the oven and roast until fragrant, about 5 minutes, tossing occasionally so they don't burn on any one side.

2. Transfer the walnuts or pecans to a large food processor fitted with the chopping blade. If you're using hazelnuts, spread them on a clean kitchen towel and set aside for 5 minutes to cool—then ball up the towel with them inside and rub it together to remove most of their papery skins. Transfer to a large food processor, leaving the skins behind in the towel.

3. Place the coriander seeds, sesame seeds, cumin seeds, peppercorns, and fennel seeds in a large skillet set over medium heat. Toast, stirring often, until fragrant, about 3 minutes.

4. Pour the spices into the food processor. Lock on the lid and pulse a couple times. Add the oil and salt; process into a grainy paste. Scrape into a bowl and serve, or store in the fridge, covered, for a few days (but let it come back to room temperature before serving).

MAKES ABOUT 8 SERVINGS

There's a cult following for these tacos across all of North America. You'll need thick-fleshed fish fillets that can be sliced like steak. Look for tortillas either in the refrigerator case of your market or in the bread aisle, sometimes fresh from a local Latin American bakery.

3 cups red cabbage, cored and shredded, or 3 cups bagged slaw mix

1 small red onion, thinly sliced

¼ cup packed cilantro leaves, chopped

¼ cup rice vinegar (see Note, page 114)

1 medium jalapeño chile, stemmed and seeded, then minced

1 tablespoon honey

1 teaspoon ground cumin

½ teaspoon kosher salt or fine-grain sea salt

½ teaspoon freshly ground black pepper

1½ pounds tuna, mahimahi, or other fish steaks

5 teaspoons sesame oil, divided

1 tablespoon chile powder

8 corn tortillas

1. Mix the cabbage, onion, cilantro, vinegar, jalapeño, honey, cumin, salt, and pepper in a large bowl. Set aside while you prepare the fish.

2. Heat a large skillet or grill pan over medium heat. Rub 1 teaspoon oil over one side of the fish, then coat it with half the chile powder. Repeat with the other side of the fish.

3. Swirl the remaining 3 teaspoons oil into the skillet or pan, then add the fish and cook until the meat inside is opaque, 7 to 9 minutes, turning once.

4. Clean and dry the skillet. Set it back over medium heat. Add the tortillas one by one, warming them up until pliable, about 30 seconds per side. Alternatively, heat the tortillas in a stack in a microwave on high for 30 seconds, then turn the stack over and heat on high for another 30 seconds. In any case, stack them on a plate, then slice the fish against the grain into long pieces. Serve all these things separately—the slaw, the tortillas, and the sliced fish—so everyone can build their own tacos at the table.

MAKES 4 SERVINGS

MAPO DOFU

Here's the dish Bruce was creating when I caught him in a state of flow (see pages 74–75). Don't be put off by the number of ingredients (or the tofu): this aromatic, Sichuan braise is terrific comfort food. By cutting the vegetables into tiny bits, you can get several in each spoonful. Serve it over brown rice for a new comfort-food favorite.

4 ounces lean ground pork, veal, or turkey

2 tablespoons soy sauce

2 tablespoons Shaoxing wine or dry sherry (see Notes)

1 tablespoon sesame oil

2 teaspoons whole Sichuan peppercorns; or 1 teaspoon black peppercorns, cracked with the bottom of a heavy skillet on a cutting board (see Notes)

8 medium scallions, root ends removed, white and green parts thinly sliced

2 medium carrots, diced

2 celery ribs, diced

3 medium garlic cloves, minced

1 tablespoon minced peeled fresh ginger or jarred preminced ginger

1 tablespoon bottled Chinese hot bean paste (see Notes)

1 cup reduced-sodium, fat-free chicken broth

1½ pounds silken firm tofu, cut into 1-inch cubes

1½ teaspoons cornstarch dissolved with 1½ teaspoons rice vinegar in a small bowl

1. Mix the ground meat with the soy sauce, Shaoxing or sherry, and sesame oil in a small bowl. Set aside.

2. Heat a large wok over medium-high heat. Add the peppercorns; toss and stir them over the heat for 1 minute.

3. Add the ground meat and all the liquid in the bowl. Stir-fry, tossing constantly over the heat with two wooden spoons, until the meat loses its raw, pink or red, color, about 2 minutes.

4. Add the scallions, carrot, celery, garlic, ginger, and hot bean paste. Stir-fry for 20 seconds.

5. Pour in the broth; stir over the heat until it comes to a full simmer. Cover, reduce the heat to low and simmer for 10 minutes.

6. Add the tofu and stir gently. Simmer for 1 minute.

7. Stir in the cornstarch mixture. Bring to a simmer, stirring gently, just until thickened, about 20 seconds. Turn off the heat, stir gently one more time, then let stand for a couple minutes to infuse the flavors.

Notes: There are three unusual ingredients in this dish.

✦ First, Shaoxing wine is a low-alcohol rice wine, found in the Asian aisle of most supermarkets. In a pinch, substitute dry sherry or even dry vermouth—or reduced-sodium chicken broth. Once opened, Shaoxing can stay in a dark, cool pantry for several months.

✦ Second, Sichuan peppercorns are the seeds from a citrus plant grown across Asia. A more esoteric ingredient, they can be found in Asian markets or from online sites. Store a bag of them in your freezer for up to two years. You can substitute fewer black peppercorns, but the taste will be less aromatic, sharper, and far less refined.

✦ Finally, hot bean paste is a fairly traditional condiment, found in the Asian aisle of almost every supermarket. Once opened, store it covered in the fridge for up to six months.

MAKES 4 SERVINGS

STIR-FRIED SHRIMP AND BROCCOLI

Most stir-fries are finished with a range of condiments that provide the depth and heft that long-cooking gives to braises. Prep all the ingredients before you begin to work over the heat. Serve this stir-fry over wilted greens, such as spinach or kale—or over brown rice.

2 tablespoons reduced-sodium soy sauce

2 tablespoons hoisin sauce (see Note)

1 tablespoon rice vinegar (see Note, page 114)

2 teaspoons honey

1 tablespoon peanut oil

4 medium scallions, thinly sliced

2 tablespoons minced peeled fresh ginger or jarred preminced ginger

2 medium garlic cloves, minced

½ teaspoon red pepper flakes

1 pound fresh broccoli florets (do not use frozen)

2 medium red bell peppers, cored, seeded, and diced (see Note, page 5)

1 pound medium shrimp, peeled and deveined (about 30 per pound—see Note, pages 19–20)

1. Whisk the soy sauce, hoisin sauce, vinegar, and honey in a small bowl until the honey dissolves. Set aside.

2. Heat a large wok or high-sided skillet over medium-high heat. Swirl in the oil, then add the scallions, ginger, garlic, and red pepper flakes. Toss and stir over the heat for a couple minutes, until the scallions have begun to soften a bit, about 2 minutes.

3. Add the broccoli florets. Stir-fry until crisp-tender, about 2 minutes. Stir in the bell peppers and shrimp. Keep tossing and stirring over the heat until the shrimp are pink and firm, about 3 minutes.

4. Pour in the soy sauce mixture; bring to a simmer. Cook, stirring constantly, a few seconds, until everything's coated.

Note: In the Asian aisle of your supermarket, look for bottlings without emulsifiers, food starches, and thickeners.

MAKES 4 SERVINGS

POMEGRANATE CHICKEN AND SQUASH STEW

This simplified version of a Persian classic should be served over couscous, a North African grain preparation. It's found near the rice or dried beans in almost all supermarkets. Buy a plain, unflavored version. The pomegranate molasses is truly the secret here, binding all the flavors and brightening them considerably.

1 tablespoon olive oil

One whole chicken, about 3½ pounds, cut into 8 to 10 pieces

1 pound frozen pearl onions, thawed

1 cup walnut pieces, chopped

1½ tablespoons unbleached all-purpose flour

1 tablespoon minced marjoram leaves or 2 teaspoons dried marjoram

½ teaspoon kosher salt or fine-grain sea salt

½ teaspoon freshly ground black pepper

2 cups reduced-sodium, fat-free chicken broth

¼ cup pomegranate molasses (see Note)

4 cups butternut squash, cubed and peeled (about 1-inch cubes)

1. Heat a Dutch oven or a heavy French casserole over medium heat. Swirl in the oil, then add the chicken, in batches, if necessary, to prevent crowding. Brown on both sides, about 8 minutes per batch; then remove to a platter and continue browning more pieces.

2. Pour off all but about 1 tablespoon oil in the pot. Stir in the pearl onions and walnut pieces. Cook, stirring often, until the pearl onions begin to brown a bit, about 4 minutes.

3. Sprinkle the flour, marjoram, salt, and pepper over the ingredients in the pot. Stir well for about 20 seconds.

4. Pour in the broth in a very slow, steady stream, stirring all the while so the flour dissolves as the broth is added. Bring back to a simmer, stirring often.

5. Pour in the pomegranate molasses; add the squash cubes. Stir well, then nestle the chicken pieces into the pot. Pour in any juices from their platter.

6. Once the sauce is at a simmer, cover, reduce the heat to low, and simmer slowly until the chicken is cooked through and the squash is quite tender, about 1 hour 20 minutes.

Note: Pomegranate molasses is pomegranate juice reduced to a thick, sweet, sour syrup and used as a basic flavoring in many Middle Eastern dishes. Look for it in the international aisle of most supermarkets.

MAKES 6 SERVINGS

SHRIMP VINDALOO

Although we think of this fiery stew as an Indian dish, vindaloo is actually Portuguese *(vinho* = wine vinegar, *ahlos* = garlic). It was introduced to the subcontinent through Goa, a trading port. Call it cultural payback: Indian cooks turned it into a fiery farrago too hot for those colonialists—except when it is pure bliss on a chilly evening. Yes, there are lots of dried spices here, but a well-stocked spice cabinet is a promise of better meals in the future. You'll be on the lookout for other recipes that will give you a return on your investment! (Like our Vegetable Biryani, see pages 51–53, or our Dried Apricot and Chicken Tagine, see pages 53–54.)

1 teaspoon kosher salt or fine-grain sea salt

½ teaspoon dry mustard

½ teaspoon ground coriander

½ teaspoon ground cumin

½ teaspoon ground ginger

½ teaspoon turmeric

¼ to ½ teaspoon cayenne pepper

¼ teaspoon ground cinnamon

⅛ teaspoon ground cloves

1½ tablespoons red wine vinegar

1 tablespoon peanut oil

1 large yellow onion, chopped

3 tablespoons minced peeled fresh ginger or jarred preminced ginger

3 medium garlic cloves, minced

1¼ cups reduced-sodium vegetable broth

2 tablespoons golden raisins, chopped

1 pound medium shrimp, peeled and deveined (about 30 per pound— see Note, pages 19–20)

1. Mix the salt, dry mustard, coriander, cumin, ginger, turmeric, cayenne, cinnamon, and cloves in a small bowl. Stir in the vinegar to create a paste.

2. Heat a large nonstick saucepan over medium heat; swirl in the oil.

3. Add the onion and cook, stirring often, until softened, about 3 minutes. Add the ginger and garlic; cook just until aromatic, no more than a few seconds.

4. Add the prepared spice paste; cook, stirring like crazy until aromatic, about 20 seconds. Stir in the broth and raisins. Bring to a full simmer; then reduce the heat to low, and simmer, uncovered, for 10 minutes.

5. Add the shrimp, raise the heat back to medium, and cook until the shrimp are pink and firm, stirring once or twice, about 3 minutes.

Note: For a great twist, serve this dish over cool cucumber noodles. To make these, take a vegetable peeler and peel a cucumber; discard these tough strips, then keep going, making long "noodles" from the vegetable as you run the vegetable peeler down its length, turning it as you go to get the flesh off every bit, right down to the seedy core. Throw this out, then start again with another cucumber. Toss the noodles with some rice vinegar and they can be a cooling bed for this fiery stew.

MAKES 4 SERVINGS

～～～～～

Build a Real Food Pantry

Since you've gotten into exploring your supermarket, it's time to start building a better pantry. Over time, of course, and within economic reason. Why? Because:

✦ You're more likely to experiment with new ingredients at the supermarket if you've got a pantry of possibilities at home—to pick up some fish you've never heard of and get it on the table by sautéing it in a little pecan oil with some dried herbs, for example.

✦ If you already have a well-stocked pantry, it won't seem so onerous to cook real food on a regular basis.

✦ A well-stocked pantry is a source of pride—and so will bring you even more pleasure through the dishes you'll make.

Consider buying a pantry staple or two every week, building up a storehouse of possibilities. As always, read those labels and remember that once opened, many condiments should be refrigerated. Here's a basic list to get you started—and keep you going!

	BASICS	LUXURIES
Oils and fats	Unsalted butter (refrigerate), a sturdy olive oil, a toasted nut oil (refrigerate), and an untoasted nut oil (refrigerate)	A delicate, high-end olive oil, toasted sesame oil (refrigerate), and avocado oil (refrigerate)
Vinegars	Rice vinegar (not *seasoned* with added sugar), balsamic vinegar, white wine vinegar, apple cider vinegar	Red wine vinegar, white balsamic vinegar, aged balsamic vinegar, and infused vinegars (beware of those with added sugars, corn syrup, or artificial flavorings)
Sweeteners	Varietal honeys, maple syrup (refrigerate), unrefined sugar	Unsulfured molasses, muscovado sugar
Whole grains	Rolled oats, long-grain brown rice, wheat berries, quick-cooking bulgur	Quinoa, wild rice, pearl barley, short-grain brown rice, medium-grain brown rice

	BASICS	LUXURIES
Ground and partially or fully refined grains	Whole wheat flour, unbleached all-purpose flour, yellow or white cornmeal	Whole wheat pastry flour (for cakes and such), wheat bran, oat bran, wheat germ (refrigerate after opening)
Dry goods and staples	Dried beans, canned beans, dried lentils, whole wheat pasta, reduced-sodium canned tomatoes, fat-free reduced-sodium chicken and vegetable broths, reduced-sodium tomato paste, baking powder, baking soda, cocoa powder, vanilla extract, no-refrigeration-needed silken firm tofu, at least one variety of shelled nut (store in the freezer)	Jarred roasted red peppers, jarred capers, rice noodles, canned low-fat coconut milk, semisweet chocolate, dried fruit (raisins, figs, and/or apricots, for example), dried chiles, dried bread crumbs
Salt and spices	Kosher salt, fine-grain sea salt, whole peppercorns (with a grinder), soy sauce, ground cinnamon, bay leaves, curry powder, dried basil, dried dill, dried oregano, dried rosemary, dried thyme, ground cumin, mild paprika, red pepper flakes, dried sage, cayenne, chile powder	Green peppercorns, Sichuan peppercorns, Asian fish sauce, caraway seeds, cardamom pods, celery seeds, dried marjoram, cinnamon sticks, whole cloves, ground cloves, dry mustard, nutmeg (buy whole and grate on a microplane), ground allspice, ground ginger, smoked paprika, sesame seeds (store in the freezer), star anise pods, turmeric
Condiments	Dijon mustard, bottled hot pepper sauce	Coarse-grained mustard, hoisin sauce, Worcestershire sauce, fruit chutney, pickled jalapeños

Finally, Take Stock

Taking the long view involves not only laying down new memory tracks for future pleasure but also knowing where you are right now. Sure, you know *what* you're eating: this peach, that fish fillet. And you may even remember it a few days later—if it was really good. But you're most likely missing out on the big picture.

Get this: people who routinely take stock of what they eat on average weigh less than those who eat without forethought.[5] To be aware is not to have less pleasure. Instead, being conscious is the way to greater pleasure—in every avenue of life!

So over the next day or two, even as you begin to open up to new foods and recipes, write down both what you eat and when you eat it. Be as precise as you can. Don't just write *a stir-fry*. Rather, write *a stir-fry with about 4 ounces of chicken, lots of broccoli, some red peppers, and a sweet/sour sauce*. If you're eating out, you may not know what went into the dish. Ask the waiter. If he or she doesn't know, do the best you can.

But before you start, here are a few ground rules:

✦ Dump any guilt or shame. Don't worry if it's not what you think it should be. Just get as complete a record as you can, taking the chart with you during the day.

✦ Don't change what you eat just because you're writing it down.

✦ Don't get demoralized. You're going to find patterns so you can improve them and enjoy food more.

✦ Consider doing this with a cohort: your spouse, friend, sibling, whomever. That said, you don't have to show each other your charts. This isn't a confessional! Following is the chart. Copy it down. Don't get obsessive, just accurate.

FOOD JOURNAL FOR

_____ **(DAY AND DATE)**

WHEN I ATE	WHAT I ATE

Our Food Journal

Bruce is sort of a nonstick guy; he avoids blame at all costs. So I sprang this journal on him one night when I casually said, "Tell me everything you ate today."

Here are our combined results:

FOOD JOURNAL FOR WEDNESDAY, MARCH 25		
WHEN WE ATE	**WHAT BRUCE ATE**	**WHAT MARK ATE**
7:00 a.m.		Breakfast at home: ½ cup homemade granola with ½ cup fat-free milk 1 large latte made with 3 shots half-caf espresso and ⅓ cup fat-free milk
8:30 a.m.	Breakfast at home: 3 pieces Whole Foods multi-grain walnut cranberry bread 2 tablespoons apricot jam 1 tablespoon natural-style peanut butter 1 large latte made with 2 shots half-caf espresso and ⅔ cup fat-free milk	
12:30 p.m.	Lunch at home: 1½ cups homemade carrot ginger soup mixed with ¼ cup cooked wheat berries 4 ounces smoked pork loin, ¾ cup purchased sauerkraut, ½ medium red-skinned potato (leftovers from dinner the night before) One large glass of seltzer with ice	Lunch at home: 1½ cups homemade carrot ginger soup mixed with ⅓ cup cooked wheat berries 3 ounces smoked pork loin, ½ cup purchased sauerkraut, and ½ medium red-skinned potato (leftovers from dinner the night before) One large glass of iced tea with lemon
1:30 p.m.	1 cup fresh-squeezed tangerine juice	

2:00 p.m.		1 small pot black tea
3:00 p.m.	Snack: one ½-inch-thick slice homemade banana bread	
5:00 p.m.	Snack: one cinnamon raisin bagel plus an iced coffee made with brewed decaf and ¼ cup fat-free milk	Snack: two ½-inch-thick slices homemade banana bread with 2 teaspoons unsalted butter
6:00 p.m.	Snack at knitting group: ⅓ cup homemade Indonesian wheat berry and carrot salad	
8:30 p.m.	Dinner out at an Italian restaurant: 3 gherkins 3 green olives 2 pepperoncini 2 wedges Italian bread One 12-inch pizza made with ⅔ cup broccoli, ½ cup boneless, skinless white meat chicken, caramelized onions in olive oil, crumbled bacon, and marinara sauce (no cheese) One 12-ounce bottle of beer	Dinner out at an Italian restaurant: 3 green olives Pasta dish with penne, Italian sausage, roasted bell peppers, caramelized onions, mushrooms, garlic, olive oil, and grated Parmesan (about 2½ cups total volume) Two 5-ounce glasses of red wine 1 mint hard candy 1 cup espresso

Just by writing it all down, we could see patterns. My caffeine intake was way up. True, I was under lots of deadlines. Still, I was downing too much coffee and tea.

And what was with the snacks? How many did we need in a day? We were eating constantly after lunch. Bruce didn't even tell me about the bagel and coffee until I pressed him. He was reticent, a sign something was amiss.

For more answers, we did a very scary thing: we sent our chart to a nutritionist. And boy, were we ever surprised at what she had to say.

Interpreting Our Chart

Joyce Hendley is everything a nutritionist should be: kind and caring, without judgment. Once the food editor for Weight Watchers publications, she's a fellow contributing editor at *Eating Well* magazine.

Here were her remarks:[6]

1. She complimented us on eating together. "So important," Joyce said, "for getting pleasure out of your meals (rather than just fueling up)."

2. She also complimented us on eating breakfast. She even encouraged Bruce's jam habit. "Jam makes breakfast feel like a treat, not dieting," she said. She also said I didn't eat enough. I never thought I'd meet a nutritionist who would tell me to eat more! "Add a piece of fruit and you'll probably be less hungry at lunch," she said. "It might be better psychologically to eat a bigger volume of food [at breakfast]—for example, have some creamy yogurt with that granola. Or what about an egg?"

3. Joyce urged us to eat more dairy. She said that we, like most Americans, are using the milk in our coffee as the dominant source of calcium. She suggested yogurt as a snack. She said our bones would thank us, especially later in life.

4. She also urged us to look more closely at how many fruits and vegetables we were eating, then increase those and complement them with occasional treats: a glass or two of wine, for example. In fact, she asked us to see more of our food choices as treats: olives, wine, beer, bagels, banana bread. "Banana bread doesn't count as fruit," she said.

5. Most of her comments were saved for our lunch— which she found too large. "Are you working in the fields?" she asked. In fact, she said that our lunch's heft

accounted for snacking in the afternoon. "A big lunch is ultimately energy-draining—it takes a lot of energy to digest that food; so unless you plan for a siesta, your energy levels will likely fade. I sense that was happening as you both tried self-medicating (Mark with banana bread, Bruce with snacks and later coffee). Self-medicating with snacks, of course, doesn't really solve the problem. Bruce was eating every two hours after lunch and mostly carb-rich foods."

6. She also advocated planning ahead. If we knew we were going to eat at an Italian restaurant, we should have had lots of veggies and even low-fat dairy during the day to balance out all the carbs in the pizza and pasta dishes. In other words, pay attention!

Interpreting Your Own Journal

Now you can spot some definite trends among your entries, using Joyce's advice as a guide.

1. Pretend for a minute that the food journal isn't yours. What dominant patterns emerge? When do you get hungry? What's your schedule?

2. What about the breads and pasta? Are you having cereal for breakfast, a sandwich for lunch, and pasta for dinner? Remember: carbs are essentially sugars. When refined (cereal flakes, white bread, white pasta), they are pretty empty of any nutrition. Are there any whole grains in your mix? (We'll come back to this in the next step.)

3. Look for the fruits and vegetables. Are you getting enough? Think of a small apple as one serving. How can you get in eight or nine of these a day? Maybe by having a plum

with breakfast, a few carrots as a snack in the afternoon. Or plan on a peach for a midmorning snack, the veggie wrap for lunch, an extra side of veggies with dinner instead of having any bread, and a small, 4-ounce glass of freshly squeezed juice in the evening as your dessert.

4. Are you giving yourself a few treats during the day? A bit of jam with that toast? Some cheese for breakfast? Don't just think sweets. Try savory pickles, olives, or a small bit of goat cheese midafternoon.

5. Watch the random eating. Notice when it's happening. Then go back to the meal before. Was it too large and so led to snacking? Or was it too small, just a salad without any variety of textures and flavors—and thus nothing really satisfying in it? Hunger can be the response to both overeating and undereating.

6. And finally, how much of the food came from your own hand? How much of it did you prepare? And how much of it was truly pleasurable?

Now Get on Schedule

Here's your taking-stock schedule for better health and more pleasure:

Once a month: keep a food journal for a day or two.
There's no need to do this every day or even every week. Instead, keep the journal, get a good take-away (*I need to eat more fruit, so I'm going to commit to a piece every afternoon as my snack*), then drop the monitoring until the next time. Soon enough, you'll find that you're eating better because you're more aware of what you're eating without being overly vigilant.

And once a week: step on the bathroom scale.
It's crucial to understanding where you are. Besides, people who weigh themselves at regular intervals statistically weigh less than those who don't.[7]

Weighing yourself can be very scary, so keep a few tips in mind:

1. Weigh yourself only once a week. Yes, there may be some weeks when your weight will fluctuate because of water retention or illness. You'll know the difference.

2. Do it at the same time every week: Thursday morning before breakfast, for example.

3. Wear similar clothing (or nothing at all!) every time.

4. Write down the number. I keep a small notebook in the bathroom with a pen nearby. Don't rely on your memory; it can get cloudy for lots of reasons.

I did it. I stepped on the scale. I didn't want to. Didn't want to so badly that I neglected, in my late forties, having a physical for three years, all because I didn't want to step on the scale at the doctor's. I was endangering my health to save a little pain.

So I did it at home. Yes, it was bad. But you know what? Within two months, I had that physical. And had already lost 22 pounds.

All because I weighed myself? Of course not. Bruce and I had begun to make better, real-food choices. But keeping track was part of it. A food journal once a month, a weigh-in once a week—these are two things that can pay off big-time.

And also make up the long view, which includes both the future (new foods you'll enjoy, new memory tracks as the basis of pleasure for future meals) and the present (where you are, what you're doing).

But notice what we didn't include: the past. Because today is the change and tomorrow is the satisfaction. Yes to all that is, and yes to all that can be. Yes, and . . .

STEP

6

Upgrade Your Choices

WHAT WILL YOU DO?
Begin to say, "Yes, and . . ." to an even
larger world
Prepare meals that pump up the nutrition
and flavor in every bite
Explore a farmers' market or
join a CSA near you

~~~~~~~~~~

WHAT WILL YOU DISCOVER?
The importance of grains, the selection, and
the best ways to get them
Ways to make selections among real food—
and add more vegetables to your choices
Seasonal eating and marketing

Be Whole

Now that you're committed to a *Yes, And* life and have begun to take stock, it's time to upgrade even more. Always push for the better alternative, buying the best you can comfortably afford.

Let's start with whole grains.[1]

I suspect I lost many of you right there.

Too bad, because the longer something is processed, the more muted its flavors, the fewer cues to satiety, the less enjoyment, the more consumption—which means we stay in our processed ruts, gaining weight without being fully satisfied.

Put simply, *refined* grains are like desserts: lovely treats, exquisitely subtle. *Whole* grains are life-sustaining.

They're the complete seeds of various grasses, rich in vitamins, minerals, protein, sugars, and fats. Every individual grain has four parts:

1. The hull. Often inedible, removed from most whole grains. If intact, the grain must often be soaked in cool water and then cooked for a long time at a low heat.

2. The bran. The hard protective outer coating underneath the hull. It holds some vitamins and minerals but is mostly stocked with fiber.

3. The germ. The tiny seed itself, what will eventually sprout into a new plant. It's got some fat, but it's mostly a wad of protein and essential nutrients.

4. The endosperm. The engine that will feed and nurture the seedling. The endosperm is a bundle of carbohydrates (a.k.a. sugars) bound up with a few proteins.

When a grain is refined, the hull, bran, and germ are removed, leaving the creamy endosperm behind. A grain of white rice is simply a polished endosperm—which acts like any other carb inside our bodies, exiting the stomach quickly to rush into the bloodstream and instigate an insulin spike before getting morphed into triglycerides and stored as fat. Why are you hungry a few hours after a Chinese dinner? Because you filled up on white rice, a big hit of carbs (along with lots of added sugars in the stir-fries).

By eating whole grains, we ingest those same, delicious, sweet carbs but also take in lots of fiber—which slows down digestion, leads to greater satiety, and buffers the inevitable spike in blood sugar. You're fuller more quickly and stay sated longer with fewer health concerns. No tough sale at all!

The bran and germ of a grain also contain significant amounts of vitamin B, a nutrient that regulates metabolism, maintains healthy skin, steadies muscle tone, and promotes cell growth—but which is depleted as we digest carbs of any kind. Eat white rice and deplete the B in your system; eat brown rice with the bran intact and replenish the B you're losing. For the nutrition we need, not to mention big flavors in every bite, we crave whole grains. With that in mind, here's our real-food chart:

REAL FOOD	ALMOST REAL FOOD	BARELY REAL FOOD	NOT REAL FOOD
Whole grains with as many of the four parts to the grain remaining as are edible	Partially refined grains (one or more of the edible parts has been removed)	Fully refined grains and flours—only the endosperm remains or is milled into flour	Instant grain products (like instant rice or polenta)

Always go for the whole-grain option when it's available. Order brown rice in a Chinese restaurant or whole-grain bread in a sandwich shop. Read through a restaurant menu to search for whole-grain options with other dishes, then ask if these can be included with your choice, or substituted for one of your sides.

However, we need to add two little warnings to our guidelines:

1. Prepared whole grains in restaurants and at food counters are often stocked with added fats and sugars so they'll quickly form a bolus (see page 15). Ask a few questions. A purer version is always preferred.

2. Many processed crackers and cereals are stocked with hydrogenated fat and high-fructose corn syrup, despite claims

of their being *an important source of whole grains.* Once again, it's all about the bolus. Read those labels to determine if you're getting a hyped fake-out.

RICE: THE LONG AND SHORT OF IT

Rice is the grain we encounter most frequently. Almost all varietals can be brown (the bran and germ in place) or white (the bran and germ removed and the kernels most likely polished for that familiar opalescence). They can be grouped into three categories:

TYPE OF RICE	COMMON VARIETALS	EXOTICS
Long grain: somewhat dry although quite fluffy, light in texture—the elongated grains do not stick together	Basmati (familiar from East Indian cooking), jasmine (very fragrant)	Carolina (the standard American long-grain varietal), patma (a favorite in India), Texmati (a cross between basmati and Carolina), black rice (sometimes called japonica), red rice (sometimes called Bhutanese rice), and pecan rice (an amber rice from Louisiana)
Medium grain: a little creamier, a little denser, even chewier—the grains stick together a bit	Arborio (familiar from risotto)	Granza, Valencia, Bomba (familiar from paella), as well as Wehani (medium-grain brown rice crossed with basmati)
Short grain: quite sticky, almost gummy—the grains clump together	Sushi rice	Hundreds of Asian varietals, most labeled as some sort of glutinous rice, sweet rice, or sticky rice

Brown rice has a rich, nutty, earthy taste. It's less sweet and thus definitely signals satiety more quickly: more flavor, more chewing, more texture, more substance. As a plus, medium-grain and short-grain brown rices are decidedly less gummy than their white counterparts.

To make the transition from white to brown rice, consider investing in a rice cooker, available at all Asian markets and online kitchen suppliers. Better models will cook any sort of rice perfectly with the mere push of a button—no need to worry about timing or heat levels.

You can also learn to love the heartiness of brown rice through one of the following three recipes, each featuring one of the varieties of this wholesome grain.

CRAB PILAF

Here's an old-school side dish turned into a main course: a casserole of brown rice with plenty of veggies and big flavors. To find long-grain brown rice, check the rice selections at your supermarket, particularly in the natural food section—or try a health-food store.

1 tablespoon unsalted butter

1 large or 2 small leeks, white and pale green parts only, halved lengthwise, washed carefully for grit, and thinly sliced (about 1½ cups)

½ pound pencil-thin asparagus spears, cut into 1-inch pieces

1½ cups long-grain brown rice, like brown basmati

2 tablespoons tarragon leaves, minced

1 tablespoon Dijon mustard

¼ teaspoon kosher salt or fine-grain sea salt

¼ teaspoon freshly ground black pepper

3 cups reduced-sodium vegetable broth

8 ounces refrigerated, pasteurized lump crabmeat, picked over for cartilage and shell

1. Preheat the oven to 350°F.

2. Melt the butter over medium heat in a large, 11-inch round, oven-safe, high-sided sauté pan or a seasoned cast-iron skillet, or in a 2-quart, flame-safe, lidded casserole. Add the leeks; cook, stirring often, until softened, about 2 minutes.

3. Add the asparagus; cook for 1 minute, stirring constantly. Dump

in the rice; continue stirring over the heat until the kernels become somewhat translucent, about 1 minute.

4. Add the tarragon, mustard, salt, and pepper, then stir in the broth. Bring to a simmer, scraping up any browned bits on the pan's or casserole's bottom.

5. Sprinkle the crab over the rice mixture, cover, and bake until the rice is tender, about 55 minutes. Fluff with a fork before serving.

MAKES 6 SERVINGS

ASIAN DIRTY RICE

Here, brown rice is paired with edamame—baby soy beans, popular in Japan, often boiled in their shells and served with a light coating of sea salt. You can find them frozen and already shelled in many grocery stores. This is a classic Louisiana recipe tilted toward Asia for a one-pot, whole-grain supper.

2 tablespoons sesame oil

1 medium yellow onion, chopped

½ pound boneless, skinless chicken thighs, cut into ½-inch pieces

⅔ cup short-grain brown rice

2 tablespoons soy sauce

2 medium garlic cloves, minced

2 teaspoons minced peeled fresh ginger or jarred preminced ginger

1⅔ cups reduced-sodium, fat-free chicken broth

1⅔ cups frozen, shelled edamame

1. Position a rack in the oven so that an oven-safe Dutch oven can fit in there with at least a couple inches of headspace.

2. Heat that Dutch oven over medium heat. Add the oil, then stir in the onion. Cook, stirring often, until translucent and softened, about 4 minutes.

3. Add the chicken thighs; cook, stirring frequently, until they've browned a bit and are frizzled at the edges, about 7 minutes.

4. Stir in the rice until it's well coated in the oil and juices; then pour in the soy sauce, garlic, and ginger. Keep stirring until the soy sauce has been absorbed.

5. Pour in the broth and the edamame. Bring to a simmer, scraping up any browned bits on the pan's bottom.

6. Cover, and bake until the rice is tender and any liquid in the pot has been absorbed, 45 to 50 minutes. Set aside covered for 10 minutes before serving.

MAKES 4 SERVINGS

GAME HENS AND RICE

Cornish game hens are small but succulent, very flavorful because the taste of the bone really gets into the meat. With chewy but moist medium-grain brown rice and lots of vegetables, this meal is a real boost of pleasure.

1 tablespoon unsalted butter

Two 1¼-pound game hens, the giblets inside removed, the birds then quartered (see Note)

1 medium red onion, chopped

1 cup medium-grain brown rice, such as brown Arborio

3 medium garlic cloves, minced

1 tablespoon minced oregano leaves or 2 teaspoons dried oregano

1 tablespoon mild paprika

2 teaspoons ground cumin

½ cup rosé wine, white wine, or water

1 large fennel bulb, the fronds and stalks removed, the bulb coarsely chopped

2 large Roma or plum tomatoes, chopped

2 cups fresh, shelled peas or frozen peas

2 cups fat-free, reduced-sodium chicken broth

½ teaspoon kosher salt or fine-grain sea salt

½ teaspoon freshly ground black pepper

1. Position a rack in the oven so that an oven-safe Dutch oven will fit in the oven with several inches of headspace. Preheat to 350°F.

2. Heat that Dutch oven over medium heat. Add the butter, let it melt, then add the game hens. Brown the pieces well, turning once (but not too soon—they need time to caramelize and release from the bottom of the pot to avoid tearing the skin off). Transfer to a plate.

3. Add the onion; cook, stirring often, until translucent, about 3 minutes.

4. Add the rice, stir about 15 seconds over the heat, then stir in the garlic, oregano, paprika, and cumin. Cook until quite aromatic, stirring once in a while, about 1 minute.

5. Pour in the wine or water; scrape up any browned bits on the bottom of the pot as the liquid comes to a simmer.

6. Add the fennel, tomatoes, and peas. Stir over the heat until the wine has been mostly absorbed into the rice and vegetables, maybe 2 minutes.

7. Pour in the broth; bring to a full simmer. Nestle the game hen pieces into the pot and pour any juice from their plate over everything.

8. Cover, place in the oven, and bake until the rice is tender, about 50 minutes. Stir in the salt and pepper. Set aside, covered, out of the oven for 10 minutes before serving so the flavors meld.

Note: To quarter game hens, cut them in half the long way, taking care that you slice on either side of the back bone (you can see it inside the large cavity). Then cut each of these pieces in half the short way, leaving a breast and wing on one and a thigh and leg on the other. Failing that butchering task, ask the person at the meat counter to do it for you.

MAKES 4 SERVINGS

A GREAT WAY TO UPGRADE: MORE AND MORE GRAINS AT EVERY TURN

Keep 'em coming. You've already met one whole grain on this journey (the bulgur in tabbouleh—see pages 47–48), but there's so much more to explore! Here are four more, with recipes to get you started.

Corn

It's easy to forget it's a whole grain, right? Right off the ear, it's a great source of thiamin (vitamin B_1), niacin (vitamin B_3), folate (vitamin B_9), vitamin C, and magnesium. The best way to get all that goodness is by having ears of corn on the cob.

PERFECT CORN ON THE COB

Since it's edible raw, cooking it is just a matter of warming it up. There's a lot of folderol in some recipes: lemon juice in the water, sugar, cook for so many minutes, don't for so many more. What's the deal? Nothing could be easier. And don't just go with the standard butter and salt on those ears. Try a little toasted nut oil and some finely grated Parmigiano-Reggiano over each.

4 ears corn

To cook them indoors: Bring a large pot of water to a boil. Meanwhile, husk the ears and pull off all the silks. Drop them in the water, turn off the heat, cover, and set aside for 10 minutes.

To grill them: Prepare the grill for high-heat cooking. Meanwhile, peel back the husks, (keeping them attached), remove the silks, press the husks back in place, and soak in water for 15 minutes. Set the ears in their husks on the grill grate directly over the heat and cook for 5 to 10 minutes, turning occasionally, until the husks are beginning to brown and even char at the edges. Cool a bit and husk before serving.

MAKES 4 SERVINGS

Wild Rice

The grain of a grass indigenous to the upper Midwest and parts of Canada, wild rice has a nutty, sophisticated taste, full of riboflavin (vitamin B$_2$), phosphorus, and potassium. One admission: wild rice takes a while to cook. Plan on forty-five minutes, maybe more depending on the grains' length. And give it lots of water—about a 1:4 rice to water ratio. The only real way to tell if wild rice is tender? Taste a grain or two. Once cooked, serve it as a side dish with butter or a toasted nut oil for flavoring; or mix it with chopped dried fruit, chopped toasted nuts, some minced veggies, a little vinaigrette, and sea salt for a salad that'll keep in the fridge for a couple days, lunch at the ready. Wild rice, dried cranberries, pecans, minced shallot, and a white wine vinaigrette make a terrific combo. You can also stuff that salad into a whole chicken or turkey before roasting either for an incredible, whole-grain treat.

WILD RICE PATTIES

Serve these as a vegetarian entrée on their own, alongside some sliced tomatoes sprinkled with sea salt and drizzled with balsamic vinegar. Or put them in whole wheat pita pockets with a creamy dressing, some chopped lettuce, and some shredded carrots.

1½ cups water

6 tablespoons wild rice

2 tablespoons walnut oil, divided

1 medium shallot, minced

6 ounces cremini or white button
    mushrooms, thinly sliced

2 tablespoons dried California
    apricots, chopped

2 teaspoons stemmed fresh thyme or
    dried thyme

½ teaspoon kosher salt or fine-grain
    sea salt

½ teaspoon freshly ground black
    pepper

1 large egg plus 1 large egg yolk

¼ cup walnuts, finely ground

1. Combine the water and rice in a small saucepan; bring to a boil over high heat. Stir, cover, reduce the heat to low, and simmer slowly until the rice is tender, about 45 minutes.

2. Drain off any excess water and transfer the cooked rice to a food processor fitted with the chopping blade.

3. Heat a large skillet over medium heat. Swirl in 1 tablespoon walnut oil, then add the shallot. Cook, stirring often, until softened, about 2 minutes.

4. Add the mushrooms; cook, stirring occasionally, until they give off their liquid and it evaporates to a glaze, about 5 minutes.

5. Stir in the dried apricots, thyme, salt, and pepper. Cook for 1 minute, then scrape the entire contents of the skillet into the food processor. Cool for 15 minutes, then pulse until finely chopped and well blended but not pureed.

6. Scrape the mixture into a large bowl; stir in the egg, egg yolk, and ground nuts until the mixture is uniform.

7. Set the skillet back over medium heat. Swirl in the remaining 1 tablespoon oil. Wet your hands, then form the wild rice mixture into four patties. Slip them into the skillet and fry until lightly browned, turning once, maybe 6 or 7 minutes in all.

Note: To grind nuts, chop them into small pieces, then place these in a large spice grinder or a small food processor. Pulse until ground to the consistency of coarse sand.

MAKES 4 SERVINGS

~~~~~~~~

Barley
A sticky grain, barley is rich in thiamin (vitamin B_1), niacin (vitamin B_3), vitamin B_6, phosphorus, magnesium, and iron. Eating barley has been shown to stabilize blood sugar levels for up to ten hours.[2] It's often served as a side dish—or added to soups and stews both to thicken them and to add a little heft (as in beef barley soup, a diner favorite.) Whole barley, available at most health-food stores, is

truly a whole grain. Even the hull is intact! To cook it, repeatedly rinse 1 cup of it in a colander set in the sink until the water runs clear. Soak the grains in cool water overnight. Drain, then sear the kernels in a large saucepan with a tablespoon of olive or walnut oil over medium heat for a few minutes, stirring constantly. Finally, pour in 3½ cups water or a reduced-sodium broth, then bring to a boil over medium-high heat. Cover, reduce the heat to low, and cook for 40 to 50 minutes, until the barley is tender. Set aside, off the heat, for 10 minutes before serving.

TOASTED BARLEY SALAD

Although whole barley is a powerhouse, most of the time we use pearled barley from the supermarket. Here, the hull is missing; thus, it's partially refined, *almost real food*—but it cooks more quickly, without any soaking, in perhaps twenty minutes. Yes, most of the vitamin B has gone missing, but the protein and other nutrients remain intact. Check the package instructions (cooking times vary with the amount of refining, although minimal in all cases). Despite being somewhat refined, pearled barley is the easiest whole-grain substitute for white rice in soups and stews (and *almost real food* is certainly better than *barely real food*). Simply stir an equivalent amount into the pot and cook the same amount of time the rice would have taken. Pearled barley also makes this healthy, nutritious salad, one that can be made ahead of time and taken to work or school for lunch.

1½ cups pearled barley (10 ounces)

1½ tablespoons olive oil

2 medium yellow onions, chopped

8 ounces cremini mushrooms, sliced

2 teaspoons minced sage leaves or
    1 teaspoon dried sage

½ teaspoon kosher salt or fine-grain
    sea salt

½ teaspoon freshly ground black pepper

¼ teaspoon ground mace

3 tablespoons cider vinegar

8 ounces grape or cherry tomatoes,
    quartered

3 celery ribs, sliced lengthwise into
    long strips, then sliced crosswise
    into small pieces

1. Position a rack in the center of the oven; preheat to 350°F.

2. Spread the barley over a large baking sheet, place it in the oven, and toast for 15 minutes, stirring occasionally.

3. Meanwhile, bring a large saucepan of water to a boil over high heat.

4. Pour the toasted barley into the boiling water. Reduce the heat to low and cook at a rolling simmer, uncovered, until tender, about 20 minutes. To tell if they're tender, scoop out a couple grains, cool a bit, and taste them. Drain in a colander set in the sink.

5. Heat a large skillet over medium-low heat. Swirl in the oil, then add the onion. Cook slowly, stirring frequently, until golden and soft, about 10 minutes.

6. Add the mushrooms, increase the heat to medium, and cook, stirring often, until the mushrooms give off their liquid and it reduces to a glaze, about 6 minutes.

7. Stir in the sage, salt, pepper, and mace. Stir for about 10 seconds over the heat, then pour in the vinegar. As it comes to a boil, scrape up any browned bits on the bottom of the skillet.

8. Scrape the entire contents of the skillet into a bowl along with the barley. Add the tomatoes and celery; toss well. The salad can be stored in the refrigerator, covered, for up to 3 days.

MAKES 6 SERVINGS

Quinoa

Described as a supergrain, quinoa *(KEEN-wah)* has the full set of amino acids, exactly those found in meat, as well as lots of thiamin (vitamin B_1), riboflavin (vitamin B_2), niacin (vitamin B_6), folate (vitamin B_9), iron, magnesium, phosphorus, and zinc. When grown, quinoa also has a natural insect repellent, saponin, surrounding each grain. However, saponin is a human-repellent, too: astringent, even bitter. Most quinoa on the market has been washed to remove the saponin, but it's still a good idea to give the grains a rinse in a colander set in the sink before cooking.

CURRIED QUINOA AND CABBAGE SALAD

If you don't want to use bottled curry powder, consider an equivalent amount of the garam masala mixture used in the Vegetable Biryani (see pages 51–53).

1 cup quinoa (about 7 ounces), rinsed

2 tablespoons peanut or almond oil

1 medium yellow onion, chopped

2 medium garlic cloves, minced

2 tablespoons minced peeled fresh ginger or jarred preminced ginger

2 tablespoons curry powder

1 teaspoon kosher salt or fine-grain sea salt

1 pound cabbage head, cut in half through the root end, thick core removed, then the leaves roughly chopped

3 tablespoons white wine vinegar

½ cup golden raisins, chopped

1. Heat a large skillet over medium heat, then add the quinoa grains. Toast them a couple minutes over the heat, stirring often.

2. Meanwhile, bring a large saucepan of water to a boil. Pour in the toasted quinoa. Cover, reduce the heat to low, and simmer until each of the grains has sprouted a translucent halo and they are tender, 12 to 15 minutes, depending on how dry the quinoa was. Drain in a fine-mesh sieve set in the sink. (Quinoa will go right through the holes of a standard colander. If you don't have a fine-mesh sieve, line a colander with cheese cloth or a large coffee filter.)

3. Set that skillet back over medium heat, then swirl in the oil. Add the onion and cook, stirring often, until translucent, about 3 minutes.

4. Stir in the garlic and ginger. Cook a few seconds, just until aromatic, then add the curry powder and salt.

5. Stir well, then toss in the shredded cabbage. Use tongs or two wooden spoons to toss it over the heat as it wilts a bit.

6. Pour in the vinegar and scrape up any browned bits on the bottom of the skillet. Cover, reduce the heat to low, and simmer slowly for 10 minutes, stirring once in a while.

7. Stir in the raisins and the drained quinoa. Toss over the heat until warmed. You can either serve the salad now or scrape it into a sealable container and store it in the fridge for up to 3 days.

MAKES 4 SERVINGS

~~~~~~

Upgrading Even Beyond Grains

If we look at our journey to real food as a whole, the first part was about making choices for foods based solely on our real food chart, avoiding *not real food*, and pushing our choices higher, toward *real food* itself. That's the sum conclusion of steps 1 through 4 of this plan.

But in the second half of this journey, we've begun defining the choices among real food itself, now starting to push out of the *barely real food* category and further into solidly *real food* territory.

In fact, even within the categories of *real food* and *almost real food*, there are choices to be made. So given what we now know about how and what we eat, let's add these two general guidelines to our established system:

✦ Eat the most of real food that's dense with nutrition but less likely to put on the pounds.

✦ Eat the least of real food that's light on nutrition and more likely to put on the pounds.

Like this:

	MORE NUTRIENTS	FEWER NUTRIENTS
Less Likely to Put on Pounds	Almost all vegetables, almost all fruits, fish, low-fat dairy, low-fat broths	Most lettuces, celery, and air-popped popcorn
More Likely to Put on Pounds	Most meat; shellfish; most casseroles; eggs; nuts and natural nut butters (without any hydrogenated oil in the mix); whole grains, including whole-grain pasta and whole-grain breads; most full-fat dairy; most cheese; honey, maple syrup, and other natural sweeteners; first-pressed and flavorful oils	Most snacks and desserts, refined sugar and other refined sweeteners, refined grains (including white rice and all-purpose flour), refined pasta, white bread, white rice (in fact, many of these would be *barely real food*—but still allowed under the general guidelines we established early on)

The bulk of what we eat should come from the upper-left-hand box. For example, if we have a steak, potato, and broccoli for dinner, the broccoli and potato should take up more of the plate than the steak. Our real food motto should always be *more veggies, please.*

We should then choose foods equally from the lower-left-hand and upper-right-hand boxes. These are also full of excellent choices; none is disallowed. But they shouldn't be the center of what we eat.

Finally, we should limit our selections from the lower-right-hand box so that we can enjoy them for the treats and specialties that they are. Yes, Bruce and I eat a lot of brown rice, but we don't love it with every Chinese stir-fry, particularly the aromatic, vegetarian ones. Occasionally, white rice fits the bill.

MORE VEGGIES, PLEASE

To renovate any of your favorite recipes, pull down the fat a bit, pull down the meat, and up the veggies or perhaps some whole grains.

Like this: a favorite recipe of creamy chicken stew has probably got great veggies like tomatoes, onions, and carrots; lots of chicken, of course; probably celery; and surely some cream and noodles. All real food—all to be relished in every bite. But how do you make a better soup, using choices among real food? By upping the veggies (more tomatoes, more carrots, more zucchini), pulling down the chicken (maybe using one thigh fewer than your recipe calls for), adding whole wheat noodles rather than refined ones (and perhaps a few less to boot), and reducing the cream to just one tablespoon per serving (replace the remainder of the liquid lost by an equivalent amount of reduced-sodium chicken broth).

Or this: when you're making a pot of long-stewed chili, cut down the meat by a bit and add some extra-long-cooking vegetables such as diced potatoes, sweet potatoes, or carrots.

It all sounds simple enough, but it can get a little complicated. First off, vegetables cook at different rates. You can't add butternut squash cubes to a quick skillet sauté and expect to have anything edible in ten minutes. If you put chopped asparagus spears into a two-hour stew, the asparagus will be disgustingly squishy.

To solve the problem, keep this chart handy so you can know what you can add when to your favorite recipes in order to up those veggies at every turn:

Quick-cooking vegetables (needing at most 15 minutes over the heat)	Asparagus, bell peppers, broccoli florets, cauliflower florets, celery, cherry tomatoes, corn, fennel, frozen or canned artichoke hearts, mushrooms, peas, summer squash, zucchini, and almost all frozen vegetables
Long-cooking vegetables (needing at least 45 minutes over the heat)	Carrots, cassava, celeriac, Jerusalem artichokes, kohlrabi, parsnips, potatoes of all stripes, rutabaga, sweet potatoes, large tomatoes, turnips, and winter squash (such as butternut, buttercup, blue Hubbard, pumpkins, and red kuri)

AN ADMISSION—WITH RECIPES

Why is it so difficult to add more vegetables? Because most require preparation.

By contrast, you buy meat ready for the skillet or oven—like strip steaks. You don't buy a full shell of beef to cut apart into individual servings at home. Instead, you buy a steak or two, already cut from that same shell.

But most vegetables come as a whole entity: a butternut squash, a beet, a carrot, an onion. By and large, they must be prepared *before* they can be cooked. No recipe asks you to plop a zucchini in a skillet! Even asparagus spears should be trimmed of their woody ends.

Here's the truth: it takes a little more time to get vegetables into your meals. Maybe it's simply a matter of recognizing the problem and facing it head-on. A little time chopping at the cutting board will make you healthier, thinner, and more satisfied. Hey, it's a great trade-off for tastes as big as these three recipes.

VEGETABLE FRITTATA

A frittata is one of the easiest meals you can imagine: an egg dish that's sort of like an omelet but without any complicated flipping. While this recipe serves only two, you can double it by using a second skillet on a second burner.

3 large eggs

2 tablespoons basil or oregano leaves, minced

½ teaspoon freshly ground black pepper

4 teaspoons olive oil

1 small yellow onion, chopped

1 small red bell pepper, cored, seeded, and diced (see page 5)

1 cup fresh peas or frozen peas, thawed

6 thin asparagus spears, woody ends removed, cut into 1-inch pieces

½ teaspoon kosher salt or fine-grain sea salt

1. Position a rack in the center of the oven and preheat to 350°F. Crack the eggs into a large bowl, add the herb of your choice and the pepper, then whisk until quite uniform, no bits of floating translucent egg white in the mix.

2. Heat a large skillet over medium heat, preferably a nonstick skillet. Swirl in the oil; then add the onion, bell pepper, peas, and asparagus. Cook, stirring often, until the onion begins to turn translucent, about 4 minutes.

3. Reduce the heat under the skillet to low. Pour the egg mixture all over the hot inside of the skillet to keep the vegetables evenly distributed. Cook for 2 minutes.

4. Set in the oven, uncovered, and bake just until the top is set, about 10 minutes. Cool in the skillet for a couple minutes, then run a heat-safe rubber spatula under the frittata to loosen it from the skillet and slide it onto a serving platter—or just cut it into halves in the skillet with that same heat-safe spatula. Sprinkle each serving with half the salt.

MAKES 2 SERVINGS

MORE-VEGETABLE-THAN-MEAT CHILI

Bruce has pulled the meat down in this traditional recipe, using it as a flavoring to make the vegetables all the more delicious. (For a similar concept, see Mapo Dofu, page 193.)

1 tablespoon olive oil

1 medium yellow onion, chopped

1 medium green bell pepper, cored, seeded, and diced (see Note, page 5)

3 celery ribs, thinly sliced

¾ pound lean pork loin or boneless, skinless turkey breast, trimmed of any exterior fat, then diced into ¼-inch cubes

⅓ cup chili powder

1½ teaspoons ground cumin

1½ teaspoons dried oregano

2 medium garlic cloves, chopped

3½ cups canned reduced-sodium crushed tomatoes (one 28-ounce can)

2 cups reduced-sodium vegetable broth

1 pound yellow summer squash, diced

1¾ cups canned kidney beans, drained and rinsed

½ teaspoon kosher salt or fine-grain sea salt

2 ounces Cheddar cheese, grated

1. Heat a large pot or Dutch oven over medium heat. Swirl in the oil. Add the onion, pepper, and celery; cook, stirring often, until the onion softens, about 5 minutes.

2. Add the pork or turkey; cook, stirring almost constantly, until it loses its raw, pink color and turns light brown, about 4 minutes.

3. Add the chili powder, cumin, oregano, and garlic. Stir over the heat until aromatic, about 30 seconds.

4. Pour in the tomatoes and broth. Bring to a simmer, scraping up any browned bits on the bottom of the pot.

5. Stir in the squash and beans; bring back to a simmer. Cover, reduce the heat to low, and simmer slowly for 1 hour, stirring a few times.

6. Uncover, stir in the salt, and continue simmering slowly until the chili thickens somewhat, about 15 minutes. After you dish it up, sprinkle a little cheese over each serving.

MAKES 6 SERVINGS

TURKEY VEGETABLE MEAT LOAF

You can even get more veggies in meat loaf? Some people make a real loaf (that is, in a loaf pan); others make *meat lump*, a mound on a baking sheet. Bruce is in the latter camp because it offers more crunchy goodness all over the outside. His recipe also includes chutney, an East Indian condiment, like a vinegary fruit jam. You can find the more run-of-the-mill mango chutney in any supermarket, but there's actually an astounding array, from tomato to blueberry, from onion to banana, at gourmet supermarkets, East Indian supermarkets, or their online outlets.

1 pound zucchini, shredded through the large holes of a box grater

3 medium carrots, shredded through the large holes of a box grater

1 teaspoon kosher salt or fine-grain sea salt

1 pound ground turkey

¼ cup fruit chutney

2 teaspoons stemmed thyme leaves or 1 teaspoon dried thyme

½ teaspoon ground cinnamon

½ teaspoon ground cumin

1 large egg

1. Toss the zucchini, carrots, and salt in a colander set in the sink. Let them sit there for 30 minutes as the salt leaches some of the moisture from the vegetables.

2. Meanwhile, position a rack in the center of the oven and preheat to 350°F.

3. Pick up the zucchini-and-carrot mixture by handfuls and squeeze tightly between your hands over the sink to remove even more water. Place these handfuls in a large bowl.

4. Stir in the ground turkey, chutney, thyme, cinnamon, cumin, and egg until everything is evenly distributed in the mixture. Gather this mixture into a ball in the bowl, then turn it out into a 9 x 13-inch baking dish. Form into a lump about like a football cut in half lengthwise.

5. Bake until an instant-read meat thermometer inserted into the thickest part of the meat loaf registers 165°F, about 1 hour.

MAKES 4 SERVINGS

～～～

A Farmers' Market: The Surest Way to Upgrade Everything You Eat

Nothing satisfies like the fresh: elemental, packed with nutrients. You respond to field-ripe blueberries, peaches, artichokes, and potatoes because, well, you're supposed to. Yes, they taste sweeter, richer, fuller; but their taste is the pleasure response to the increased nutrition. It's a perfect cycle: stimulus and reward, no fake-outs at all.

Almost everything at a farmers' market fits into our *real food* category—with the possible exception of a few jams and jellies that would drop into the *almost real food* box. If you're serious about real food, then you're going to get serious about farmers' markets because you'll find organic chickens, farmstand cheeses, ripe strawberries, and supersweet butternut squashes.

As of last count, there are 4,685 across the United States, up 6.8 percent in just two years. To find one near you, ask around or check out www.localharvest.org.

WHAT MAKES A FARMERS' MARKET DIFFERENT FROM YOUR LOCAL SUPERMARKET

For the most part, farmers' markets mean one thing: locally grown food. The green market in Manhattan's Union Square dictates that the goods can have traveled no more than 200 miles. Some markets in less intensely urban settings have even stricter rules. After all, there's little sense in buying an organic lemon at a farmers' market in Minneapolis, a lemon that has traveled thousands of miles, using up gallons of gasoline, when in fact that self-same organic lemon can be found at a similar price at a local supermarket where it has shared the gas cost with a truckload of other produce.

At a farmers' market, you can shake the hand of the man or woman who actually grew the produce or raised the lambs. You're more connected with your food—and where it comes from. You're also proud of your purchases: you hunted for it, found it, and got the best there is. That all adds up to more-pleasurable, less-processed fare.

As you wander the stalls, sampling fresh produce and deciding what's going to end up on your plate tonight, look for

1. Long Lines
There's no reason to reinvent the wheel. The old-timers know which stalls are best through trial-and-error.

2. Dirt

That's a sign that the veggies have come right out of the ground. Washing off a little grit at home is a small price to pay for exquisite taste.

Also be prepared to ask a few questions, like:

✦ *What kind of apple (or peach or cheese) is this?* Even if it doesn't really matter, it's good to see if the person selling the item is informed.

✦ *How do I pick a good one?* Watch out for answers like, *They're all good.* Of course they are. You want to hear back things like, *Well, when do you want to eat it?* or *What are you going to use it for?*

✦ *When did you pick this?* This is a way to see if the person growing the produce is in fact the person you're dealing with.

✦ *What pest control do you use?* We asked this once of a woman at the Dane County Farmers' Market in Madison, Wisconsin, and got this answer: "Our hands—we pick off the bugs and pull the weeds ourselves." We knew right then we were standing at the table of a farmer who really cared for her produce.

✦ *How do you care for the soil?* You'll hear more than you may want to know, but you'll also learn a lot about your food.

FARMERS' MARKETS USE A SLIGHTLY DIFFERENT VOCABULARY, TOO

You'll see all sorts of signs that describe what you're buying. Here are some words that have specific meanings in this real-food context:

Conventional

Standard, modern, agricultural technology, methods, pesticides, and/or hybridization are in use on the farm.

Natural

A term without teeth, it means nothing *unnatural* was added to, used on, or administered to the produce, meat, cheese, or what have you. However, a vast horde of food additives, pesticides, herbicides, and fungicides can be counted as *natural* since they arose from chemical and physical processes that occur (or once occurred) in nature.

Pesticide-free

The farm probably doesn't use synthetic pest-killers, fungicides, or herbicides. However, it may still use synthetic fertilizers. Ask pertinent questions to find out more.

Organic

Crop rotation, composting, and/or hand cultivation have been used extensively without any synthetic fertilizers or pesticides. Anything labeled *organic* must have been certified by approved USDA organizations (unless the individual farm has less than $5,000 a year in annual sales).

Transitional

Most transitional farms use organic practices but have not yet passed the required three-year waiting period for full certification.

Vine-ripened or tree-ripened

The fruit was fully ripe before it was picked. Many commercial fruits are picked green, then shipped long distances; some (for example, tomatoes) are artificially ripened with gasses.

Farmstand produce

The farmer who raised the food is selling it. Farmstand cheeses come from milk produced on the very farm where the cheeses are made, not from milk shipped in from other farms.

Free-range

The USDA regulates this term only for poultry—and only stipulates that the birds have access to the outdoors for a brief period of time. In other words, a small cubbyhole of a door can be opened in a huge barn for fifteen minutes every day, the birds rarely venturing out, and they can then all be labeled *free-range*. It's best to talk to farmers directly.

Grass-fed

The cows or pigs were fed only fresh pasture grasses in the spring and summer, then dried hay the rest of the year or during periods of drought. The animals may or may not have access to the outdoors.

Antibiotic-free

The animals were not given needless antibiotics. However, they may have been given drugs when sick. That said, fewer than 10 percent of the more than 26 million pounds of antibiotics administered yearly to animals is given to prevent actual diseases.

Hormone-free

The animals were not given hormones to increase their size, their milk production, or other factors. *Organic* does not necessarily mean *hormone-free*, for not all hormones are synthetic.

As you learn the lingo and stroll among the producers, you'll also find out ways to cook all that farm-fresh produce. Talk to the growers. They know best. Keep exploring, investigating, and learning. This way lies true pleasure.

Getting Even Closer to the Farm—and More Serious About Real Food: A CSA

If you're really committed to real food, you'll want to join a CSA (that is, Community Supported Agriculture). Here's how it works: you buy shares in a farm, then reap the harvest during the growing season.

We belong to Chubby Bunny, a CSA in Falls Village, Connecticut, that produces a bounty of produce from June to early November. Bruce and I buy a half share and get more produce each week than we can eat: for example, a couple pounds of salad greens, zucchini, cucumbers, melons, radishes, corn, acorn squash, potatoes, garlic. In the end, we're more connected to the season because we know what's coming in from the harvest.

If you live in a city, many CSAs have drop-off points in urban areas. Ours has a weekly delivery to Manhattan's Upper West Side.

However, CSAs can be pricy. Our half share is $350. True, that's a onetime payment, spread out over twenty-three weeks (or about $15 a week, or a little more than $2 a day). It's less than we would pay for organic produce at a farmers' market, but the up-front, lump payment is no doubt a hit. Ask if your fee can be divided out over time. Or split a share (or even a half share) with a friend.

To find a CSA near you, check out www.localharvest.org or contact your state's department of agriculture.

HOW TO EAT SEASONALLY

As you frequent farmers' markets and maybe even join a CSA, you begin to compose your meals based on the seasons, pushing real food to the very best it can be: fresh, right off the vine or tree, full of flavor and almost no processing. You've come so far in your journey, away from the fake stuff that rules so many lives and has contributed to an obesity epidemic of undersatisfied people.

Of course, the seasons change with longitudes and altitudes; however, this reference guide and a few recipes will point you in the right direction. Find your season now and consider making its best produce a part of your meals in the days ahead.

Summer
Summer is the time when the berries and large stone fruits shine: raspberries, blackberries, blueberries, as well as peaches, nectarines, and plums. It's also the time of great watermelons. To pick the best, just turn them over and look at the pale spot on the underside: if it's fully beige, the watermelon is ready to eat (if it's white or brown, the watermelon was picked too soon or too late). Summer's also full of tomatoes, leafy greens, eggplant, squash, zucchini, corn, and potatoes. Don't waste a minute of it!

PANZANELLA

This traditional Italian salad made from day-old bread and ripe tomatoes is summer in a bowl. Buy the freshest, ripest tomatoes you can find and use them that very day without ever putting them in the refrigerator.

A long, thin loaf of stale, day-old bread, preferably a crusty loaf like a baguette, cut into 1-inch cubes (about 2 cups)

½ pound green beans, cut into 1-inch pieces

1 medium garlic clove, minced

3 tablespoons red wine vinegar

½ teaspoon fine-grain sea salt

½ teaspoon freshly ground black pepper

¼ cup very fragrant olive oil

16 ounces (1 pound) cherry tomatoes, cut in half

1 medium cucumber, peeled, cut in half lengthwise, the seeds scooped out to be discarded, and then the flesh thinly sliced

1 small red onion, diced

1. Preheat the oven to 350°F. Spread the bread cubes on a large baking sheet, then toast them in the oven until brown and a little crunchy, tossing occasionally, 15 to 20 minutes.

2. Meanwhile, bring a small pot of water to a boil over high heat. Add the sliced green beans; cook for 1 minute, then drain them in a colander set in the sink.

3. Whisk the garlic, vinegar, salt, and pepper in a large serving bowl. Whisk in the olive oil in a slow, steady stream; continue whisking for 20 seconds.

4. Add the green beans, tomatoes, cucumber, and red onion; toss well. Add the cubed bread, toss gently, and serve at once.

MAKES 4 SERVINGS

Frozen spinach bears almost no resemblance to delicate, sweet fresh spinach in the summer. And many of us don't really know it. It's time to get more familiar with this summer marvel. The cheese and pine nuts in this rich pie will offer a nice bit of protein without any added meat.

6 phyllo sheets, thawed according to the package instructions

2 teaspoons olive oil, plus more for brushing the dish and phyllo dough

1 small yellow onion, chopped

2 medium garlic cloves, minced

16 ounces (1 pound) fresh spinach, thick stems removed, the leaves washed but not dried

¼ cup packed oregano leaves

2½ ounces finely grated Parmigiano-Reggiano

1 large egg

1 teaspoon finely grated lemon zest

½ teaspoon red pepper flakes

¼ teaspoon grated nutmeg

¼ teaspoon fine-grain sea salt

3 tablespoons golden raisins, chopped

3 tablespoons pine nuts

1. Position a rack in the center of the oven and preheat to 350°F. Set the phyllo sheets on a cutting board, cover with plastic wrap and then a clean kitchen towel.

2. Heat a large skillet over medium heat. Swirl in 1 teaspoon oil, then add the onion and garlic. Cook, stirring often, just until the onion starts to turn translucent, about 2 minutes.

3. Add the spinach; toss well. Cover, reduce the heat to low, and continue cooking, tossing often, until the spinach is wilted and the skillet is mostly dry, about 5 minutes. Pour into a large food processor. Cool for 10 minutes.

4. Add the oregano, grated cheese, egg, lemon zest, red pepper flakes, nutmeg, and salt. Pulse several times to form a grainy paste; then add the raisins and pine nuts and pulse one or two times to combine.

5. Lightly brush the inside of a 9-inch square baking dish with some of the remaining olive oil. Set one phyllo sheet in the baking dish, centered so it laps evenly over two sides. Brush the sheet very lightly with oil, then add a second sheet, this time perpendicular to the first sheet. Brush this second one very lightly with oil—in fact, from now on, brush every added sheet with a little oil. Add a third sheet, this time at a diagonal to the other two sheets, then a fourth perpendicular to the third. Finally, add the last two sheets in the same direction as the first two. Press the sheets down so they adhere to the contours of the baking dish and cover its inner surface.

6. Spoon and scrape the spinach mixture into the baking dish. Fold the hanging-over edges of the phyllo sheets on top of the pie. They won't cover it completely; instead, they'll give it a decorative edging.

7. Bake until the phyllo is brown and crunchy and the filling is hot and set, about 40 minutes. Cool on a wire rack for 10 minutes before cutting and serving.

MAKES 4 SERVINGS

〜〜〜〜〜〜

Autumn

One of the best things about early autumn is that you've got the last of the summer plenty even while the days are getting cooler. Apples and pears, with their complex flavors and delicate sweetness, are a farewell to the fading summer, a last hurrah. The roots and hard squashes are also starting to come in: parsnips, turnips, butternut squash, pumpkins, and the rest. These hearty vegetables can make a last stand for abundance before we hunker down.

BROILED HADDOCK WITH VEGETABLE NOODLES

You'll need a vegetable peeler to make long "noodles" out of the zucchini and yellow squash. Their textures and flavors add up to lots of satiety in this simple meal. Want even more? Add some mashed potatoes on the side.

2 large zucchini

2 large yellow squash

2 tablespoons olive oil

12 ounces cherry tomatoes, halved

1 tablespoon rice vinegar or white wine vinegar (see Note, page 114)

½ teaspoon kosher salt or fine-grain sea salt

½ teaspoon freshly ground black pepper

Four 6-ounce haddock fillets

½ cup fresh bread crumbs (see Note)

¼ cup mixed fresh herbs, such as thyme, basil, tarragon, parsley, or sage, minced

1 large lemon, quartered

1. Use a vegetable peeler to make long "noodles" from the zucchini and yellow squash, running it down the length of the vegetables to create long strips, then turning the vegetables to make more strips along different areas, stopping when you reach a large seedy core.

2. Heat a large skillet over medium heat. Swirl in the oil, then add all the vegetable "noodles." Toss and stir over the heat just until they begin to soften, about 2 minutes. Add the tomatoes and cook for another minute.

3. Take the skillet off the heat, then stir in the vinegar, salt, and pepper. Divide this mixture among four serving plates.

4. Position a rack about 5 inches from the heat source and preheat the broiler.

5. Set the haddock fillets on a large, lipped baking sheet; then set the sheet on the rack and broil for 3 minutes.

6. Meanwhile, mix the bread crumbs and herbs in a small bowl.

7. Use a large spatula to turn the haddock fillets, then top them with the bread crumb mixture. Baste with any juices on the baking sheet, then squeeze a lemon quarter over each fillet, taking care not to knock off the topping.

8. Continue broiling until the bread crumbs have browned a bit, about 3 minutes. Set one fillet on top of each bed of noodles on the plates.

Note: Fresh bread crumbs are made from *fresh* (if stale) bread. To make them yourself, cut part of a baguette or other crunchy loaf into slices and leave them out on the counter overnight. Process the pieces in a food processor until they're like coarse sand. Or go to almost any supermarket's bakery and buy a bag of fresh bread crumbs there. They'll keep, sealed tightly, in the freezer for a couple of months.

MAKES 4 SERVINGS

~~~~~~~

BEST-EVER POT ROAST

If you've got company, this hearty autumn supper can be doubled for crowds. Ask the butcher to help you pick out a good chuck roast, one without too much fat.

1¼ pounds beef chuck roast

½ teaspoon kosher salt or fine-grain sea salt

½ teaspoon freshly ground black pepper

1 tablespoon unsalted butter

1 large yellow onion, halved and thinly sliced

4 medium yellow-fleshed potatoes, such as Yukon Golds, halved

1 medium celeriac (a.k.a. celery root), any roots or fuzz removed, peeled, then cut into 1-inch cubes

1 small butternut squash, peeled, halved lengthwise, seeds removed, and cut into 1-inch cubes

2 medium garlic cloves, minced

1 cup dried cranberries

¼ cup bottled white horseradish

1 cup reduced-sodium, fat-free chicken broth

1. Position a rack in the oven so that a Dutch oven will fit in there with at least 3 inches of headspace. Preheat the oven to 325°F.

2. Season the roast with salt and pepper. Melt the butter in that Dutch oven over medium heat. Add the beef and brown really well on both sides, about 8 minutes in all.

3. Transfer the beef to a plate, then add the onion. Stir over the heat just until it turns translucent, about 3 minutes.

4. Stir in the potatoes, celeriac, butternut squash, and garlic. Cook for 2 minutes, stirring all the while; then stir in the cranberries.

5. Nestle the meat into these vegetables, spreading them to the sides so it sits evenly on the bottom of the pan. Slather the horse-radish over the top surface of the beef. Pour the broth around the meat so as not to knock off the horseradish coating. Bring to a simmer.

6. Cover and set in the oven. Bake until the meat is falling-apart tender, about 2½ hours. Cool in the pot for 10 minutes before cutting into bits and serving with the broth and veggies.

MAKES 4 SERVINGS

Winter

Although winter seems harsh, it has its bright spot: citrus. Lemons, limes, grapefruits, kumquats—these are little shards of light during darker days. It's also the time for the *keeping vegetables*: rutabagas, onions, leeks, broccoli, Brussels sprouts, and other sturdy, hearty things that can stand up to cellaring and storing while we wait the coming of the fuller light.

SOUTHWESTERN CHICKEN BRAISE

The sweet potatoes in this mix will add the perfect balance to the spiky heat, brought on by the combination of a jalapeño's sour spark and the more complex heat of chile powder. In fact, chiles are a great way to spike up a wintry dish (not to mention the ways they add up to more satiety more quickly—see pages 102–103).

1 small yellow onion, quartered

2 large garlic cloves, halved
    lengthwise

1 pickled jalapeño chile, stemmed

2 tablespoons chile powder

2 teaspoons ground cumin

½ teaspoon kosher salt or fine-grain
    sea salt

1 tablespoon almond, pecan, or
    sesame oil

2½ pounds boneless, skinless chicken
    thighs, cut into 1-inch cubes

One 12-ounce dark Mexican beer

1 large rutabaga, peeled with a
    vegetable peeler, then cut into
    1-inch cubes

1 tablespoon honey

One 4-inch cinnamon stick

1 tablespoon yellow cornmeal

1. Place the onion, garlic, jalapeño, chile powder, cumin, and salt in a food processor fitted with the chopping blade or a mini food processor; process until a thick paste. If you don't have a food processor, you can cut the onion into eighths, set all these ingredients on a large cutting board, and repeatedly rock a large chef's knife through them until they're pasty, repositioning them constantly so they keep falling under the rocking blade until they make a similarly thick paste.

2. Heat the oil in a large Dutch oven over medium heat. Add the chicken and brown well on all sides, turning occasionally, about 6 minutes.

3. Stir in the spice paste and cook until quite aromatic, about 3 minutes.

4. Pour in the beer, add the rutabaga cubes, and scrape up any browned bits on the pot's bottom. Add the honey and cinnamon stick. Bring to a simmer; cover, reduce the heat to low; and simmer slowly for 1 hour, until the rutabaga cubes are tender.

5. Stir in the cornmeal; simmer, uncovered, stirring often, until somewhat thickened, about 10 minutes.

MAKES 6 SERVINGS

ROASTED BROCCOLI AND CAULIFLOWER WITH PASTA AND CHEESE

This is one of our favorite dinners: a wintry casserole of roasted vegetables, tossed with pasta and cheese. It's got fiber, protein, carbs—the works. In other words, real food in every bite. A vinegary salad afterward makes the meal complete.

12 large garlic cloves, unpeeled
(see Note, page 184)

4 cups cauliflower florets

4 cups broccoli florets

2 tablespoons olive oil

2 ounces thinly sliced prosciutto,
chopped

½ cup reduced-sodium canned
vegetable broth

1 tablespoon stemmed thyme leaves

½ teaspoon red pepper flakes

8 ounces dried whole wheat pasta
mini shells or orecchiette, cooked
and drained according to the
package's instructions

¼ cup dry white wine

2 ounces grated Parmigiano-
Reggiano

2 tablespoons minced chives or the
green part of a scallion

½ teaspoon freshly ground black
pepper

1. Position a rack in the center of the oven and preheat to 425°F.

2. Place the garlic cloves in a 9 x 13-inch baking dish. Bake for 20 minutes.

3. Add the cauliflower florets, broccoli florets, and olive oil. Toss well with a couple wooden spoons or heat-safe spatulas. Reduce the oven's heat to 400°F. Continue baking the vegetables for 20 minutes, tossing and stirring a couple times. Transfer the baking dish to a wire rack and cool for a few minutes, just until you can handle those garlic cloves.

4. Squeeze the soft garlic pulp out of its papery hulls and back into the baking dish. Stir in the prosciutto, broth, thyme, and red pepper flakes. Stir well, and continue baking for 10 minutes.

5. Transfer the baking dish back to the wire rack. Stir in the pasta, wine, cheese, chives or scallions, and pepper. Toss just until the cheese melts, then serve while hot.

MAKES 4 SERVINGS

Spring

Pay attention to the asparagus and peas, harbingers of life coming back from the earth. Then be ready for apricots and cherries, rhubarb and strawberries. As a special treat, look for black or red currants, sour bits of early sunshine, best in a pie or crisp—or even in a sauce for duck or pork. Later in the spring search out carrots, radishes, and cherry tomatoes, all sure signs that the sun is again gaining force and life is very good.

PEA AND RADISH SALAD WITH FETA

This early-season salad would be a welcome addition alongside a piece of fish off the grill—or even a rotisseried chicken from the supermarket. There are so many flavors in this simple salad that it'll force you to slow down and savor them.

3 cups shelled fresh peas	1½ tablespoons lemon juice
8 medium radishes, halved and thinly sliced	1 tablespoon oregano leaves, chopped
⅔ cup crumbled feta	1 tablespoon dill fronds, chopped
1½ tablespoons olive oil	2 teaspoons honey

1. Bring a large pot of water to a boil over high heat. Add the peas and cook for 2 minutes, stirring occasionally. Drain the peas in a colander set in the sink, rinse under cool water, then shake dry and dump them into a large bowl.

2. Add everything else to that bowl and stir well before serving.

MAKES 4 SERVINGS

CHICKEN CACCIATORE

Although it seems like a cool-weather stew, cacciatore is a dish that looks to spring because of all the fresh vegetables. In fact, Bruce has made this version even more springlike with fresh cherry tomatoes. Pancetta is an unsmoked, cured bacon, often sold rolled into logs at the deli counter. Don't buy it paper-thin and presliced; instead, buy a chunk at the deli counter, then dice it at home, for a better bit of texture and flavor in the stew.

1 tablespoon olive oil

2 ounces pancetta, diced into small cubes

4 bone-in chicken thighs

1 medium yellow onion, chopped

1 medium carrot, diced

1 medium green bell pepper, cored, seeded, and diced (see Note, page 5)

½ pound green beans, cut into 1-inch pieces

1 pound cremini mushrooms, thinly sliced

⅔ cup red wine, or fat-free, reduced-sodium chicken broth, or a combination of both

1 pound cherry tomatoes, diced

2 teaspoons stemmed thyme or 1 teaspoon dried thyme

1 teaspoon finely grated lemon zest

½ teaspoon freshly ground black pepper

Kosher salt or fine-grain sea salt, to taste

1. Heat a Dutch oven or a heavy French casserole over medium heat. Swirl in the oil, then add the pancetta cubes. Cook, stirring occasionally, until frizzled at the edges and lightly browned, about 4 minutes.

2. Use a slotted spoon to remove the pancetta from the pot and

transfer the pieces to a plate. Add the chicken thighs. Cook, turning once, until well browned on all sides, about 5 minutes. Also transfer these to that plate.

3. Add the onion, carrot, bell pepper, and green beans. Cook, stirring often, until the veggies begin to soften, about 5 minutes.

4. Stir in the mushrooms. Cook, stirring often, until they give off their liquid and it reduces to a glaze in the pot, about 6 minutes.

5. Stir in the wine and/or broth, then scrape up any browned bits on the bottom of the pot as the liquid comes to a full simmer. Continue simmering until the liquid is half its original volume, about 2 minutes.

6. Stir in the tomatoes, thyme, lemon zest, and pepper, as well as the pancetta, the chicken thighs, and any juice on their plate. Bring to a simmer; then cover the pot, reduce the heat to low, and simmer until the chicken is quite tender and the tomatoes have broken down into a sauce, about 1 hour. Although the pancetta is salty, you might find you want to add a few extra sprinkles of salt to individual servings.

MAKES 4 SERVINGS

7

Treat Yourself Well

WHAT WILL YOU DO?

Have a better breakfast

Combat midday hunger

Finish up with dessert

~~~~~~~~~~

WHAT WILL YOU DISCOVER?

A few last warning signs,
but even more tips for success

Three ways to pamper yourself

Start Here: Eat Breakfast

There are lots of reasons we miss the first meal of the day: getting the kids off to school, too much work, and too little sleep. But eating breakfast is a prime way to tell if you're treating yourself well:

✦ Breakfast regulates the insulin levels in your bloodstream. Over time, those dips and spikes are a root cause of a host of ailments, including heart disease.[1]

✦ Breakfast brings up your glycogen levels, leading to more glucose (or brain food) in your system. If you regularly skip breakfast, you're probably also sluggish in the mornings.

✦ Skipping breakfast means you're more likely to pick high-fat, high-calorie foods during the rest of the day, up to 200 calories worth.[2] Your body is desperate to compensate.

So start the day off right with some real food. Breakfast may well be the easiest place to get some whole grains—with a boxed, whole-grain cereal, topped with milk or yogurt and a piece of fruit alongside. Here are a few tips for picking the right cereal:

1. If you see any hydrogenated shortening in the ingredient list, put the box back on the shelf. We've already discounted hydrogenated shortening as *not real food*. No need to put it back on the table now.

2. The very first listed ingredient should be a whole grain. If you see a milled grain, cornmeal, or even flour on the list, you aren't getting what you think you're getting.

3. Also look for added sugars, even corn syrup or fruit juice concentrates (which are a form of sugar). Grains are already full of carbs; there's little reason to fill them up with excess calories.

We recently found a so-called natural granola on the market that had this as its stated ingredient list:

+ *whole-grain rolled oats,*

+ *evaporated cane juice,*

+ *pineapple juice concentrate,*

+ *pear juice concentrate,*

+ *peach juice concentrate,*

+ *vitamin E (a natural vitamin to help preserve flavor),*

+ *natural flavor.*

Yes, a whole grain starts the list; but by our count, there are four sources of sugar. No wonder each serving (shy of half a cup!) has 12 grams of sugar—or 3 teaspoons—and comes in at 200 calories. (And we're not even mentioning whatever that *natural flavor* is.)

There's no doubt about it: breakfast is a tough spot for real food mavens. We crave carbs—sugars, most of all—because they jump-start our brains (and even our digestive systems). But by doing a little investigating in the ways we've already learned, we can get more flavor in every bite, more real food at every turn. Once again, don't discount convenience; instead, evaluate it.

Of course, you might want to go even further. Following are three whole-grain, make-ahead breakfast recipes that'll let you treat yourself right every day and still cut your time in the kitchen when you're trying to get out the door. But try to keep in mind what you learned early on: don't eat on the run. Have some coffee, spend some time on a social networking site, or catch up on the morning's news. Life is busy. It needn't be insane.

REFRIGERATOR MUFFINS

This is an old-fashioned idea: a whole-grain batter made in advance, then stored in the fridge for a few weeks. Each morning, bake off as many muffins as you'd like. One note: there's no standardized size for muffin tins. This recipe was designed for tins that hold ½ cup in each indentation.

2 cups organic raisin bran cereal

1¼ cups boiling water

½ cup oat bran cereal

1½ cups low-fat buttermilk

¾ cup sugar, preferably unrefined, raw sugar

6 tablespoons honey

6 tablespoons walnut oil, plus more for pan

1 large egg plus 1 large egg white

2 cups whole wheat flour

2 teaspoons baking soda

1 teaspoon ground cinnamon

½ teaspoon fine-grain sea salt

1. Mix the raisin bran cereal, boiling water, and oat bran in a large bowl. Set aside at room temperature for 10 minutes.

2. Stir the mixture until smooth (except for the raisins in the cereal, of course), then stir in the buttermilk, sugar, honey, and walnut oil.

3. Stir in the egg and egg white; then, finally, stir in the flour, baking soda, cinnamon, and salt until there are no pockets of undissolved flour lurking anywhere, particularly in the bottom of the bowl.

4. Scoop the batter into a resealable container, then refrigerate for at least 24 hours or up to 1 month.

5. To bake the muffins, preheat the oven to 375°F. Rub a little walnut oil into as many muffin indentations in a pan as you intend to make, taking care to get it into the place where the bottom seams against the side. Fill the indentations about three-quarters full, then bake the muffins until a toothpick inserted into the center of one comes out with a few moist crumbs attached, 20 to 25 minutes.

MAKES 18 MUFFINS

MULTIGRAIN WAFFLE MIX

Now you're ready to go for a weekend breakfast.

FOR THE DRY MIX

1½ cups unbleached all-purpose flour

1½ cups whole wheat flour

⅔ cup yellow cornmeal

½ cup toasted wheat germ (see Note, page 164)

¼ cup turbinado sugar, maple sugar, or other unrefined sugar

2 tablespoons baking powder

2 teaspoons salt

FOR THE BATTER (3 WAFFLES)

1 large egg

2 tablespoons toasted nut oil

½ cup low-fat milk, plus more as needed

1. Combine all the dry mix ingredients in a resealable plastic container; store at room temperature for several months.

To make 3 waffles: Mix 1 cup plus 2 tablespoons of the mix with the egg and nut oil. Add the milk and stir well. Because flour holds moisture based on humidity, you might have to add a little more milk to make a batter. But remember: waffle batter is slightly thicker than pancake batter. Heat the waffle iron and make the waffles according to the manufacturer's instructions.

MAKES 12 WAFFLES

MUESLI

This no-cook breakfast will set your morning off right. It must be made ahead of time, then stored in the fridge, a meal at the ready.

2 cups rolled oats (do not use quick-cooking or steel-cut oats)

1¾ cups regular or low-fat plain yogurt

1½ cups cranberry or pomegranate juice

½ cup dried cranberries, chopped

1 tablespoon honey

2 teaspoons vanilla extract

Mix the ingredients in a resealable container. Cover and refrigerate overnight. The muesli can be stored in the fridge for 1 week.

MAKES 6 SERVINGS

Then Do This: Snack Appropriately

Midafternoon most days, you probably start to flag, your concentration a little off, your mood a little flat. It's inevitable. You've been running around all day. And the time between lunch and dinner is just too big.

If you're not just flagging but getting overtly hungry, you may be facing one of two problems:

1. *You may have eaten too much or too little for lunch.* A cheeseburger, fries, salad, and dessert is simply too much unless you plan on resodding your lawn. Likewise, a handful of baby carrots and a diet soda will not hold you till dinner. As we've already learned, hunger is often the response to both overeating and undereating. If you find yourself plagued with tummy gurgles by midafternoon, go back and do a basic food journal for a couple days, just to check your patterns. And don't just assume that you ate too much at the meal before. We knew someone who complained of midafternoon snacking because she'd had a sausage roll at a farmers' market. Sure, there are lots of calories there, but it might actually be too little food: too little variety, too little fiber, too little protein. She'd probably have been more content if she'd had her roll with some spicy radishes, then enjoyed a crisp apple afterward.

2. You may not be sleeping enough. There's definitive research that a lack of shut-eye is directly correlated with snacking. A group of people were followed through their days after having their sleep time cut to about 5½ hours a night. While they did not consume more at mealtimes, they certainly upped their intake of high-calorie, high-carbohydrate snacks.[3] In truth, we're all sleeping less these days, down to about 6.1 hours a night on average.[4] Your first defense against snacking may well be a good night's sleep, about 8 hours. That's definitely treating yourself right!

Still and all, assuming you're not getting legitimately hungry but just flagging midafternoon, you can still find it hard to resist the temptation to start snacking with candy machines, break rooms, stocked refrigerators, bodegas, and a bevy of 100-calorie snack packs at every turn.

Mindless, between-meal eating remains the way most of us consume food—and the most empty calories, to boot—without much thought, without tasting or chewing. A 100-calorie cupcake in an individually wrapped package isn't going to bring any satisfaction to the game. Chances are, it's not even going to bring great taste. That's not treating yourself very well. That's not real food.

A better strategy is to have a piece of fruit midafternoon. Make sure you have grapes, oranges, peaches, figs, or blueberries at home or at work. If they're in the fridge or in your desk, you're more likely to reach for them, rather than something processed from the pantry or vending machine—particularly if you make that piece of fruit a true treat with a cup of tea or coffee on the side. Think of it as a little meal. In fact, see it that way.

Or try one of these alternatives to the processed and packaged 100-calorie snacks:

✦ A handful of whole wheat pretzels with some spicy mustard

✦ 1 ounce soft goat cheese spread on a piece of crunchy bread

✦ 1 ounce feta drizzled with 2 teaspoons honey and lots of freshly ground black pepper, along with a couple of all-grain crackers such as FinnCrisps

✦ Apple wedges with natural peanut butter—or better yet, honey mustard

✦ A medium orange and a few dry-roasted nuts

✦ A few dried apricots and a handful of salted pistachios

✦ ½ cup low-fat yogurt mixed with a handful of berries and a teaspoon or two of honey

✦ Eight or so black olives warmed in a microwave with some grated orange zest

✦ A ripe pear with ½ ounce blue cheese

✦ An avocado half, sprinkled with lemon juice and salt—or with jarred salsa

✦ Frozen grapes. Store green or red grapes in the freezer; pull them out in about ½ cup servings, little bites of ice cold bliss, like sucking candies, only much better

✦ Carrot sticks with about 1 ounce soft goat cheese

✦ A small, 5-ounce baked potato (you can cook it in the microwave—or the night before when you're making dinner) topped with a little salsa

✦ About ½ cup unsweetened applesauce—or a little less with a slice of whole wheat toast

✦ 2 large graham cracker squares with 1 teaspoon peanut butter and some low-fat milk

✦ A quarter of a 2- to 3-ounce bittersweet or semisweet pure chocolate bar

Or to treat yourself really well, try one of the following three recipes for midday treats:

PARMESAN CRISPS

These are just crispy rounds of fried cheese. The first one or two may take a little practice, but you'll soon get the hang of it. And keep in mind they're a great treat when friends drop over. (Just make more for generosity's sake!)

5 tablespoons Parmigiano-Reggiano grated with the small holes of a box grater or a cheese microplane

Freshly ground black pepper

1. Heat a large nonstick skillet or well-seasoned cast-iron skillet over medium-high heat.

2. Drop little nests of finely grated Parmigiano-Reggiano in 1-tablespoon increments into the skillet. Grind a little black pepper on each.

3. The cheese will immediately begin to melt, spread out, and bubble fiercely. Drop the heat to medium but do nothing else. Eventually, the melting cheese will form an irregular circle that starts to caramelize. Once it's deeply golden, scoop it up out of the skillet with a nonstick-safe spatula. The little disk will be bendy and limp. You can straighten it out as you transfer it to a wire rack—but be careful, it's quite hot. Cool until crunchy, about 1 minute. And have at them.

MAKES 5 CRISPS
(JUST A SKOSH OVER 100 CALORIES)

GRANOLA

While it's a great breakfast, granola is also a terrific afternoon snack. This recipe will make a lot—because you can store it sealed at room temperature for up to two months. For a treat around 100 calories, scoop out about ½ cup and take it with you as a midafternoon snack in a small plastic bag.

6 cups rolled oats (do not use steel-cut or quick-cooking oats)

½ cup powdered dry fat-free milk

½ cup toasted wheat germ (see Note, page 164)

¼ cup almonds, walnuts, or skinned hazelnuts, finely chopped

¼ cup muscovado sugar

1½ teaspoons ground cinnamon

1 teaspoon fine-grain sea salt

½ cup maple syrup

½ cup almond or walnut oil, plus a little additional for greasing the baking trays

1 tablespoon vanilla extract

½ cup raisins or other dried fruit, chopped

1. Position the racks in the top and bottom thirds of the oven. Preheat the oven to 325°F.

2. Spread the oats on two baking sheets. Place in the oven; bake for 5 minutes. Stir the oats, then spread them out flat. Reverse the trays top to bottom and back to front. Continue baking another 5 minutes. Transfer to a rack to cool for 5 minutes.

3. Pour the oats into a large bowl. Mix in the powdered milk, wheat germ, nuts, muscovado sugar, cinnamon, and salt.

4. Mix the syrup, oil, and vanilla in a small saucepan. Heat over medium-low heat just until warm, with some puffs of steam off the mixture.

5. Pour the syrup mixture over the oat mixture and stir well with a wooden spoon. Dab a little oil on a crumpled paper towel and lightly grease the two baking sheets. Spread the oat mixture evenly onto these baking sheets (remember: they'll still be hot).

6. Bake for 10 minutes, then stir the granola on the sheets, flattening it back out evenly across the sheet. Reverse the sheets back to front and top to bottom. Continue baking until lightly browned and quite aromatic, about another 10 minutes.

7. Transfer the sheets to a wire rack. Stir half the raisins or dried fruit into each sheet, then spread the mixture flat again and cool to room temperature, at least 2 hours. Break up, pour into a large container, and seal tightly.

MAKES TWENTY-TWO
½-CUP SERVINGS

THREE POPCORN SPICES

Forget boring popcorn! Here are a few spice mixtures that'll make enough for a batch or two of popcorn from a hot-air popper.

SOUTHWESTERN POPCORN SPICE

2 teaspoons chile powder

1 teaspoon ground cumin

1 teaspoon paprika, preferably smoked paprika

½ teaspoon garlic powder

½ teaspoon fine-grain sea salt

HERBED PARMESAN POPCORN SPICE

3 tablespoons finely grated Parmigiano-Reggiano

2 teaspoons dried thyme

½ teaspoon garlic powder

¼ teaspoon fine-grain sea salt

GREEK-STYLE POPCORN SPICE

1 tablespoon dried dill

1 tablespoon dried lemon peel, ground

½ teaspoon fine-grain sea salt

To make any of these, simply mix them together and store them in a resealable container at room temperature for up to 1 week. Each makes enough for 6 to 8 cups of air-popped popcorn.

And Finally: Eat Your Dessert

We've said all along that treats should be treats. If we've eaten a cupcake here, a candy bar there, all several times during the day, how do we know they're treats?

Consider one sweet a day your limit. Otherwise, there's that hideous taste-deadening that goes on with too much sugar, a condition we've tried to rid by detoxing out palates.

Still, who can argue with the wonders of good desserts? So how do you balance your choices?

Make only as much as you intend to eat. There's no need to make three dozen cookies if you're the only one eating them. If you're craving a three-layer chocolate cake, make sure you have enough people to share it with. (Bring it to work or church and make lots of friends!)

All along, we've stressed the importance of making meals events, of eating them with people. Desserts and sweets are a very good place to take stock. If you find yourself eating sweets alone most of the time—in front of the TV at night or in the car on your way to your errands—there's probably a problem afoot. You may be using those sweets as a way to soothe jangled nerves or other uncomfortable feelings. Besides, you're probably not getting full satisfaction from them.

And that's too bad because your relationship with them is the essence of our plan. Eating them alone robs them of most of their pleasure.

So save your sweets for when you're with friends, relatives, company. Enjoy desserts as celebratory food. And real food, for sure—so long as you forget the fake at every turn. (There's no better test case for *that* than sweets and desserts.) And so long as you keep in mind that they're not to be constant and certainly not tranquilizing. Sweets and desserts are fairly empty calories, certainly in the lower-left-hand box in our pounds/nutrients chart (see page 224). There's no reason to have too many. But there's also no reason to avoid them. So go for it! Here are four that certainly fit the bill in our real-food chart.

RASPBERRY CRISP

One way to make sure you make only the amount you can eat is to make crisps and such in muffin tins. Use one with indentations that hold about ½ cup. You'll instantly know what a serving size is. Now that's treating yourself right! Want to take this dessert over the top? Pour on a little honey-sweetened yogurt.

3 cups fresh raspberries

¼ cup unrefined sugar

1 tablespoon instant tapioca

¼ teaspoon fine-grain sea salt, divided

¼ cup unbleached all-purpose flour

¼ cup rolled oats (do not use steel-cut
or quick-cooking oats)

3 tablespoons muscovado sugar

2 tablespoons sliced almonds

2 tablespoons walnut or almond oil

1 tablespoon maple syrup

¼ teaspoon ground cinnamon

1. Position a rack in the center of the oven and preheat to 350°F.

2. Mix the raspberries, unrefined sugar, tapioca, and ⅛ teaspoon salt in a large bowl. Divide among 6 ½-cup muffin tin indentations.

3. Mix the flour, oats, muscovado sugar, almonds, oil, syrup, cinnamon, and the remaining ⅛ teaspoon salt in a large, clean bowl. Sprinkle this mixture evenly over the raspberry mixture in the indentations.

4. Bake until lightly browned and bubbling, about 25 minutes. Cool on a rack for at least 10 minutes—or cool to room temperature, then cover the tin with plastic wrap and store at room temperature for up to 2 days.

MAKES 6 SERVINGS

BUTTERMILK BROWNIES

Once again, the muffin tin gives us the right portion. These are light, moist, and intensely chocolate. What more do you need? A glass of milk, of course.

Walnut oil or another nut oil, for
greasing the tins

¼ cup unbleached all-purpose flour

6 tablespoons natural cocoa powder

¼ teaspoon baking soda

¼ teaspoon fine-grain sea salt

¼ cup regular or low-fat buttermilk

6 tablespoons unrefined sugar

1 teaspoon vanilla extract

1. Position a rack in the center of the oven and preheat to 350°F. Pour a little oil onto a wadded-up paper towel and lightly grease 6 ½-cup indentations in a muffin tin.

2. Mix the flour, cocoa, soda, and salt in a bowl.

3. In a second bowl, whisk the buttermilk, sugar, and vanilla until the sugar dissolves.

4. Use a wooden spoon to stir in the flour mixture until a batter forms and all pockets of undissolved flour are gone.

5. Divide among the prepared indentations, about 2 tablespoons in each. Bake until set and fairly firm to the touch, about 15 minutes. Cool in the tin for 5 minutes, then transfer to a rack and cool completely. When completely cooled, store in a resealable plastic container at room temperature for up to 2 days.

MAKES 6 SERVINGS

CHEWY WALNUT CHOCOLATE COOKIES

Bruce has developed this recipe so that you don't end up with three dozen cookies on the counter. These are like little meringues that remain chewy and light after being baked in a low-heat oven.

A nut oil, parchment paper, or a
   silicon baking mat
½ cup muscovado sugar
3 tablespoons well-beaten egg (a little
   less than 1 large egg)
¾ ounce unsweetened chocolate,
   chopped and melted in a small
   saucepan over very low heat or in
   the microwave, then cooled

½ teaspoon vanilla extract
6 tablespoons unbleached all-purpose
   flour
3 tablespoons walnuts, chopped
¼ teaspoon baking soda
⅛ teaspoon fine-grain sea salt

1. Position a rack in the center of the oven and preheat to 250°F. Lightly grease a large baking sheet with oil or line it with either parchment paper or a silicon baking mat.

2. Beat the muscovado sugar and egg in a large bowl until creamy with an electric mixer at medium speed, about 3 minutes, scraping down the sides of the bowl with a rubber spatula occasionally.

3. Beat in the chocolate and vanilla. Turn off the beaters; add the flour, walnuts, soda, and salt; then beat at low speed just until the flour has dissolved, not much more time than half a minute perhaps.

4. Drop by tablespoonfuls onto the prepared baking sheet, sort of like big Hershey's Kisses. Bake until set and a little firm on the outside (although soft inside), about 1 hour 15 minutes.

MAKES 12 COOKIES (OR 4 SERVINGS)

CHOCOLATE CHUNK–OATMEAL COOKIES

When Bruce was developing recipes for this book, he brought a little bag of these to lunch with friends. One friend later confessed she hoarded her share and ate them one at a time over three days. Now *there's* someone who knows how to relish real food!

4 tablespoons (½ stick) unsalted butter

6 tablespoons unrefined sugar

1 tablespoon well-beaten egg

1 teaspoon vanilla extract

½ cup plus 1 tablespoon rolled oats
    (do not use steel-cut or quick-
    cooking oats)

¼ cup plus 1 tablespoon unbleached
    all-purpose flour

¼ teaspoon baking soda

¼ teaspoon ground cinnamon

¼ teaspoon fine-grain sea salt

⅔ cup bittersweet chocolate, chopped

1. Position a rack in the center of the oven and preheat to 375°F.

2. Beat the butter and sugar in a large bowl with an electric mixer at

medium speed until creamy and light, about 3 minutes, scraping down the sides of the bowl occasionally with a rubber spatula.

3. Beat in the well-beaten egg and vanilla until smooth.

4. Turn off the beaters; add the oats, flour, soda, cinnamon, and salt. Beat at low speed until a batter forms, no more white pockets of flour anywhere, maybe just 15 seconds. Stir in the chocolate chips.

5. Roll the dough into 12 balls about the size of golf balls. Place them on a large baking sheet a few inches apart, then flatten slightly with the palm of your hand or the back of a wooden spoon, just until the sides crack a bit.

6. Bake until firm and set, about 16 minutes. Cool on the baking sheet for 5 minutes, then transfer to a wire rack to continue cooling. Once at room temperature, the cookies can be sealed in a plastic container and stored at room temperature for up to 2 days.

MAKES 12 COOKIES (OR 4 SERVINGS)

A Fond Farewell!

It's been a great journey—but the next part is even better: a life of pleasure. How can you make sure that will happen?

Keep investigating real food.
There's so much more to learn: organic practices, sustainability issues, artisanal producers, new foods from new countries. You could spend the next month just investigating the world of cheese at your farmers' market or from producers you can find in your area by a simple Web search. You'll find a host of artisanal products at sites like americanfeast.com—or do searches for specific things that interest you: wine, jams, jerky, beef, pork, or even produce. You can also start to learn about the problems with factory-farmed meat, the issues with overfishing certain ocean stocks. Keep exploring, looking at food blogs, and checking out cookbooks. Real food is a passion. It sustains life. It makes it better. It's worth the time you put into it.

Bring back dinner parties.
Reinvigorate the practice of having family and friends over for full meals. After all, you've got all this real food on the table! A multi-course affair on a Saturday night over a bottle of wine and lots of laughter is a blessing beyond compare.

Keep exploring the world.
There are supermarkets aplenty all around. Find new ones, if only because you'll see things outside your routine. Or go further: plan vacations around some food destinations like Montreal, Paris, San Francisco, Vancouver, Barcelona, or New York City. Or go all out and take a food tour of a region of the country—or even abroad. Look at tasteofspain.com for some ideas. Even on a road trip in your home state, investigate food finds along the way: search out cheese makers or bakeries before you leave, making it a point to stop by and see what's up. Bruce and I always head out with a list of farmers' markets near our destination. And when we teach cooking classes aboard Holland America Line cruises, we never leave home without a list of markets we want to check out, a collection of reservations at local restaurants, and some ideas about where to find the best artisanal products in the countries we're visiting.

Never take real food for granted.
Celebrate our plentiful gifts at every turn. Find fresh fruit and berries every summer; enjoy them as the juice runs down your chin! This is life at its essence, a way not only to become healthier and thinner, but a way to open yourself up to the crazy, beautiful, redemptive world. You'll find yourself more loving, more accepting, happier, and more satisfied. We've lived too long with our guts in an uproar, horrified with this political movement or that economic catastrophe. It's time to sit down at the table and relish real food. It's time to celebrate life.

Be well, be healthy, and find yourself immersed in the thick of things. Don't stand back. Pick up your fork and dig in. *Bon appétit! Tutti a tavola a mangiare!* いらっしゃいませ! Let's eat many more peaches!

Acknowledgments

A book is like dinner: the effort of two people in the kitchen obscures the work of legions.

This book had not one but two terrific editors. After acquiring it, Cara Bedick worked tirelessly to straighten out our Henry James moments, caught in logic and sentences that defied gravity. More than anything else, the book reflects her keen-eyed clarity and graceful intelligence. Tricia Boczkowski then worked tirelessly to keep us afloat through the editorial process after the words got on the page and in the right order. She has never been a whit less than professional, personable, and smart—a miracle combination. These two are simply amazing.

After eighteen books and fourteen years, it's hard to even comprehend the work of our agent, Susan Ginsburg. We wouldn't have a career without her. She instantly believed in the original proposal for this book (*Diets Suck!*) and then saw it through the tangle of multiple offers and contract niceties. And after all that, she still brought us the best nougat from Paris!

She could because Bethany Strout has made things run so smoothly in the office at Writers House. Many thanks to her for opening up breathing room in this rather breathless business.

We've wanted to work with Nisha Sondhe for years—and can't believe we landed a book where her urbane photographer's schedule finally meshed with our laid-back country life. We had so much fun taking all the shots at our house with her and her superb assistant, Eric Medsker. We can only hope all our paths continue to cross.

At Gallery Books, we owe deep gratitude to a roll call of often-unsung heros: Dan Cabrera, the editorial assistant; Jaime Putorti, the book's designer; Michael Nagin, the jacket designer; Michelle Lomuscio, the production manager; Alexandre Su, the production editor; Jennifer Weidman, the senior counsel for the house; and Kate Dresser, who kept the busy business of details from overwhelming us.

Also at Gallery, Kristin Dwyer has tirelessly overseen the book's publicity push (we loved her from that first meeting!). Andrea Peabbles was a terrific, savvy copy editor, catching the remaining flaws after we got done with the thing.

Finally, this book, more than any other we've ever written, owes an enormous debt to some brilliant recipe-testers: Dale Brown (ever the best), Heidi Finan (loved that bare honesty), Beth Thorman (a family to feed from new recipes—a wonder indeed!), Sarah Mroue (a terrific palate), and Steve Albert and Carter Inskeep (such sheer enthusiasm). What's here is a direct reflection of their takes and tastes—exacting eyes for real food, nothing less. We cannot thank them enough.

Endnotes

Welcome!

1. E-mail correspondence with Leslie Fink, April 4, 2009. Satiety will prove an important concept in our journey. It means a state of being sated, of being full and content, definitely not stuffed, but well fed and happy.

2. In July 2009, the U.S. Centers for Disease Control released its disturbing obesity statistics: no state in the United States has an obesity rate lower than 19% (Colorado's rate—and apparently a bit of good news, if you can count an obesity rate of slightly less than one out of every five people as good news). Seventeen states, clumped mostly in the West and New England, had rates below 24%. The rest had rates above 25%, with six states cresting 30% or better. In Mississippi, almost one in three people are obese. And we're not talking overweight, a separate category with its own CDC numbers. Obesity is defined as having a body mass index greater than 30—for example, if you're 5 foot 9 and weigh more than 203 pounds. For more information on this problem, check out the CDC's factsheets at www.cdc.gov/obesity/data/trends.html.

3. Allison A. Hedley, et al., "Prevalence of Overweight and Obesity Among U.S. Children, Adolescents, and Adults, 1999–2002," *The Journal of the American Medical Association*, vol. 291, no. 3 (2004), pp. 2847–2850.

4. Statistic cited from the Associations' website factsheet at www.restaurant.org/aboutus/faqs.cfm.

5. We're talking about the people most likely to buy this book, not some universal *we*. In truth, many people do not have enough to eat. Yes, globally, of course. For that story, see Roger Thurow and Scott Kilman's *Enough: Why the World's Poorest Starve in an Age of Plenty* (New York: PublicAffairs, 2009). But closer to home, too. In the United States, some of us go hungry every day. According to the United States Department of Agriculture's latest statistics, more than 36 million Americans (including more than 12 million children) do not know where their next meal will come from. That figure represents more than 11% of the population. (And it came from a 2007 study, at the height of the good times, before the economic meltdown.) If you go to a public park in a U.S. city, chances are that slightly more than one in ten of the people you see go hungry some of the time.

6. That is, *have a good meal* in French, *everyone to the table to eat* in Italian (a phrase popularized by TV Chef Lidia Bastianich), and *irasshaimase (ear-ahsh-eye-mahs*—that is, *come in*, the Japanese greeting yelled at you when you enter a sushi restaurant).

Step 1: Learn the Secrets to Satisfaction

1. Mostly via dopamine, a powerful neurotransmitter, common across a huge spectrum of life on this planet, vertebrates to invertebrates. Dopamine has many functions, including stimulating voluntary movement (see a fly and swat it away, thanks in part to dopamine); but its most pressing function for us right now is its ability to set up reward-based pleasure. For more information, see K. C. Berridge, "Food Reward: Brain Substrates of Wanting and Liking," *Neuroscience and Biobehavioral Reviews*, vol. 20, no. 1 (1996), pp. 1–25; and K. C. Berridge and M. L. Kringelbach, "Affective Neuroscience of Pleasure: Reward in Humans and Animals," *Psychopharmacology*, vol. 199, no. 3 (2008), pp. 457–480. For a more detailed examination of the mechanism by which dopamine works in the brain as a food reward, see M. F. Roitman, et al. "Dopamine Operates as a Subsecond Modulator of Food Seeking," *Journal of Neuroscience*, vol. 24, no. 6 (2004), pp. 1265–1271.

2. B. C. Wittman, et al., "Reward-Related fMRI Activation of Dopaminergic Midbrain is Associated with Enhanced Hippocampus-Dependent Long-Term Memory Formation," *Neuron*, vol. 45, no. 3 (2005), pp. 459–467.

3. For the link between memory and pleasure, see R. A. Adcock, et al., "Reward-Motivated Learning: Mesolimbic Activation Precedes Memory Formation," *Neuron*, vol. 50, no. 3 (2006), pp. 507–517; and B. Knutson and R. A. Adcock, "Remembrance of Rewards Past," *Neuron*, vol. 45, no. 3 (2005), pages 331–332.

4. See, for example, A. K. Anderson and N. Sobel, "Dissociating Intensity from Valence as Sensory Inputs to Emotion," *Neuron*, vol. 39, no. 4 (2003), pages 581–583.

5. Particularly as stress sets in. We feel bad under stress, then we eat and feel better, not because the stress was relieved but because the reward chemicals in the brain are naturally released from food consumption—except we've made a false, coincidental connection between stress relief and eating. For more information, see M. F. Dallman, et al., "Chronic Stress and Obesity: A New View of 'Comfort Food,'" *Proceedings of the National Academy of Sciences of the United States of America*, vol. 100, no. 20 (2003), pp. 11696–11701.

6. For depressing evidence that we can eat just to eat, see N. D. Volkow and J. S. Fowler, "The Role of Dopamine in Motivation for Food in Humans: Implications for Obesity," *Expert Opinion on Therapeutic Targets*, vol. 6, no. 5 (2002), pp. 601–609; and C. Clantuoni, et al., "Evidence That Intermittent, Excessive Sugar Intake Causes Endogenous Opioid Dependence," *Obesity Research*, vol. 10, no. 6 (2002), pp. 478–488; as well as M. S. Jog, et al., "Building Neural Representations of Habits," *Science*, vol. 286, no. 5445 (1999), pp. 1745–1749.

7. Of course, this advice doesn't take into account the problems of the compulsive eater, someone who eats far beyond the norm, someone who simply cannot stop once started. The best plan available—and a nice pairing with our real-food steps—is the one started by Overeaters Anonymous. Check out meeting locations via the various sites on the web.

8. There are even overtones based on other senses, a deep connection to the world around us, like rain, tides, leather, grass, roses, violets, oaks, smoke, and even earth.

9. Without a doubt, the best indictment of this romanticized food past is Susanne Freidberg's *Fresh: A Perishable History* (Boston: Belknap Press, 2009). Freidberg takes apart the notion that *fresh* is somehow a neutral concept, as if we ever really ate much that could be considered fresh anyway. (The concept of *fresh* may well be a marker of class status, not necessarily a truth about the food we eat.) Maybe when we go out to our garden, pick a tomato, and savor that wonderful taste, maybe then we're actually eating *fresh*. But only then. Not otherwise at the supermarket, nor even at the farmers' market. Everything else is hours, days, even weeks away from the farm. And so it's gone for the many millennia of cured meats and vinegary vegetables, especially in those long epochs before anyone even thought of refrigeration. Whenever Bruce and I hear some finger-wagging locavore proclaim that she or he would never eat anything frozen, we always think about what our options would be in the dead of winter in rural New England. Compromise is the essence of life. Ideals are both our salvation and our damnation.

10. For the complete story of how our jaws shrank and cooked food kick-started human civilization, see Richard Wrangham's *Catching Fire: How Cooking Made Us Human* (New York: Basic Books, 2009).

11. See E. T. Rolls and J. H. Rolls, "Olfactory Sensory-Specific Satiety in Humans," *Psychology and Behavior*, vol. 61, no. 3 (1997), pp. 461–473. As the authors say

in their conclusion: "[S]low eating, by allowing olfactory and gustatory sensory-specific satiety time to build up, may tend to reduce meal size" (p. 472).

12. From Harvard Medical School and University of Minnesota studies cited in Amanda Hesser's "Commander in Chef," *New York Times*, May 30, 2009.

13. For an excellent history of how beef came to its current state of production and consumption, see Andrew Rimas and Evan Fraser's *Beef: The Untold Story of How Milk, Meat, and Muscle Shaped the World* (New York: William Morrow, 2008).

14. Just to do the calorie count for a second, our lunch at home even with the beers came to about 540 calories. The cheeseburgers at the restaurant—with no fries—ran about 900 calories. And if we'd gone for a more loaded burger, say with bacon and guacamole, and even had the fries to boot, we'd have neared 1,600 calories—almost the full amount of calorie intake anyone needs for a day.

Step 2: Make Informed Choices

1. No one's better on the topic than Jean Baudrillard, especially in *Simulacra and Simulation*, trans. Sheila Faria Glaser (Ann Arbor: University of Michigan Press, 1994). He argues that our world is awash in simulacra—that is, simulations that make reality claims. These particular simulations are not pudding per se, but they become it over time, when enough of us have ceased to remember what real pudding is.

2. This may be the first time you've read the nutritional information from a food product label. The ingredients are listed in a decreasing order of *weight*. The first thing on the list is *by weight* the biggest part of the package. However, weights can be tricky. A cup of granulated white sugar weighs less than a cup of water (219 grams for the sugar; 227 grams for the water).

3. See www.fda.gov/Food/FoodIngredientsPackaging/ucm115326.htm.

4. Paul Roberts, *The End of Food* (New York: Houghton Mifflin Harcourt, 2008), p. 47.

5. From Alissa Hamilton's *Squeezed: What You Don't Know About Orange Juice* (New Haven: Yale University Press, 2009), p. 35.

6. Susan E. Swithers and Terry L. Davidson, "A Role for Sweet Taste: Calorie Predictive Relations in Energy Regulation by Rats," *Behavioral Neuroscience*, vol. 122, no. 1 (2008), pp. 161–173. As the authors state: "The data clearly indicate that consuming a food sweetened with no-calorie saccharin can lead to greater body-weight gain and adiposity than would consuming the same food sweetened with a higher-calorie sugar."

7. For the complete story, see www.foodnavigator-usa.com/Science-Nutrition/FDA-re-opens-probe-into-benzene-contamination-of-soft-drinks. For more

information on the whole problem of labeling and nutrition, see Marion Nestle's *Food Politics: How the Food Industry Influences Nutrition and Health* (Berkeley: University of California Press, revised and expanded edition, 2007). Also check out Kelly D. Bonnell's *Food Fight: The Inside Story of the Food Industry, America's Obesity Crisis, and What We Can Do About It* (New York: McGraw-Hill, 2003).

8. Some may object to the sugar and chocolate in the pudding. Both are definitely refined. But one step at a time. We're not going to lose either. But we're eventually going to modify them a bit.

9. From Alissa Hamilton's *Squeezed: What You Don't Know About Orange Juice* (New Haven: Yale University Press, 2009), p. 35.

10. Our serving sizes had to be adjusted from those given on the packages. The one for the natural fish fillets was quite a bit lower than those for both the store brand and our own—about 85% of the total weight of our haddock fillets. So we pulled the data on the natural fillets up to an equivalent amount of food as compared to the other two categories in our experiment (thus, eating 15% more of the fish sticks to get the equivalent amount of food as we would from the homemade fillets).

11. Bruce counted the oven's preheating in the complete timing. However, while it came up to its constant temperature of about 400°F, he prepared our fish fillets. In other words, he was working on ours while the oven was preheating.

12. Data from the USDA's Economic Research Service: Eating and Health Module (ATUS), 2007 Table 6. www.ers.usda.gov/Data/ATUS/Data/2007_table6.htm.

13. Mihaly Csikszentmihalyi, *Flow: The Psychology of Optimal Experience* (New York: HarperPerennial, 1990), p. 71.

Step 3: Relish What You Eat

1. That's Swanson's Hungry Man XXL Dinner, Roasted Carved Turkey. The calorie information is provided by The Calorie Counter at www.caloriecount.about .com/calories-swanson-hungry-man-xxl-dinner-i115944.

2. We're eating a lot of frozen dinners, too: on average, six a month. From "Frozen TV Dinners—A Cornerstone of the American Diet," Fooducate Blog, April 6, 2009, www.fooducate.com/blog/2009/04/06/frozen-tv-dinners-a-cornerstone-of-the-american-diet.

3. The actual number of calories consumed by the average American has jumped from 2,231 calories per day in 1970 to 2,757 calories per day in 2003. All these statistics were compiled from "U.S. Food Consumption up 16 Percent Since 1970," *Amber Waves: The Economics of Food, Farmings, Natural Resources, and Rural America* (United States Department of Agriculture Economic Research

Service, November 2005), http://www.ers.usda.gov/AmberWaves/November05/Findings/USFoodConsumption.htm. One note: while dairy consumption did increase marginally, the amount of calories consumed through dairy actually went down (about 11%), thanks in large part to the growth of the low-fat dairy market.

4. The story is told fully in Nicolette Niman's *Righteous Porkchop: Finding a Life and Good Food Beyond Factory Farms* (New York: Collins Living, 2009).

5. For a review of the current diet literature, see Julie Moynihan and Maggie Villiger's terrific article "Do Diets Work?" on pbs.org at www.pbs.org/saf/1401/features/diets.htm. The writers follow two Danish researchers who figure out that of the nine hundred studies to prove the truth of various diet plans in the thirty years prior to 2000, only seventeen used accurate scientific methodology. The rest were sheer hucksterism.

6. Mireille Guilano, *French Women Don't Get Fat: The Secret of Eating for Pleasure* (New York: Knopf, 2004).

7. In fact, French obesity rates are climbing quickly. By 2020, the French will most likely have caught up to Americans. See Elaine Sciolino, "France Battles a Problem That Grows and Grows: Fat," *New York Times*, January 25, 2006.

8. Aristotle was one of the first to articulate a pleasure factor at the heart of human behavior. He called his fundamental necessity of human existence *happiness (eudaimonia*, a state of well-being based on personal success and enjoyment of the world) in the *Nicomachean Ethics*, particularly in Book 1 and then again in Book 9. The best contemporary study may well be Norman Bradburn's *The Structure of Psychological Well-Being* (Chicago: Aldine Publishing Company, 1969). Bradburn posits that happiness is a state distinct from unhappiness—that the two are in fact not linked and that happiness is instead linked directly to pleasure as a motivating principle.

9. More pleasure, more good nutrition, too. There was a now-famous study conducted in the mid-1970s in which Thai and Swedish women were fed spicy Thai meals of rice and vegetables, laced with hot chiles, coconut milk, and stinky fish sauce. The Thai women relished the food—and surprisingly absorbed more iron from the food than the Swedish women. Not a little more iron, but a lot—almost 50% more, in fact. The experiment was then reversed and the same women were fed Swedish, meat-and-potatoes meals. Now the Swedish women relished the food and absorbed more iron, the Thai women lagging behind by as much as 70%. And then one more thing: the Thai meal was put in a blender, whirred up into an appalling goo, and fed to those Thai women. Same meal as before, hideous consistency. Now the Thai women absorbed much less iron as they complained about the nasty stuff they were supposed to drink. In all these cases, enjoyment appears to have affected nutrient uptake. In other words, if we like something, our brains may send signals to our guts to slurp it up. If we don't, our bodies

quite literally pass. (Sorry—bad pun.) For a more detailed analysis of this study and what it means to our diets, check out Barry Glasner's *The Gospel of Food: Everything You Think You Know About Food Is Wrong* (New York: Ecco, 2007).

10. There was a 2004 survey by *Parade Magazine* that found that people had stopped worrying about carbohydrate consumption altogether and were in fact eating more carbs than ever, despite the still-incessant blather in the media about the necessity of no-carb, high-protein diets. You can watch *Parade's* food editor Fran Carpentier discuss the matter on CBS' The Early Show at www.cbsnews .com/stories/2004/11/11/earlyshow/health/main655224.shtml.

11. These stats come from Raj Patel's *Stuffed and Starved* (New York: Melville House Publishing, 2007), p. 289. Statistics from the United States Department of Labor are slightly different if nonetheless corroborative. According to the U.S. government, the average American man spent 4 minutes a day shopping for food and 15 minutes a day preparing it, consuming it, and cleaning up after it; the average American woman, 8 minutes shopping and 47 minutes preparing, consuming, and cleaning up. See the November 2005 issue of the Department of Labor's *Amber Waves: The Economics of Food, Farming, Natural Resources, and Rural America* found at www.ers.usda.gov/AmberWaves/November05/ DataFeature.

12. The stat comes from a 2008 NDP study quoted in Amanda Hesser's "Commander in Chef," *New York Times*, May 30, 2009.

13. Diane Troop, "Glacial Growth for Frozen Dinners" at FoodProcessing.com, www.foodprocessing.com/articles/2006/158.html.

14. Stats from Stacy Hunt's "Getting Off the Professed Food Conveyor," *Celsias*, www.celsias.com/article/getting-off-the-processed-food-conveyor; and "Global Packaged Food: From Added Value to Availability," in *Euromonitor International*, www.euromonitor.com/Global_packaged_food_from_added_value_to_ availability.

15. Julia Child, et al., *Mastering the Art of French Cooking*, volume 1 (New York: Knopf, 1961), pp. 241 and 224.

16. L. R. Young and M. Nestle, "Expanding Portion Sizes in the U.S. Marketplace: Implications for Nutrition Counseling," *Journal of the American Dietetic Association*, vol. 103 (2003): pp. 231–234.

17. Jenny H. Ledikwe, Julia A. Ello-Martin, and Barbara J. Rolls, "Portion Sizes and the Obesity Epidemic," *American Journal of Nutritional Sciences*, vol. 135 (April 2005), pp. 905–909.

18. Phone call with Barbara J. Rolls, July 30, 2009.

19. "How Much Time Do Americans Spend Preparing and Eating Food?" *Amber Waves: The Economics of Food, Farmings, Natural Resources, and Rural Amer-*

ica (United States Department of Agriculture Economic Research Service, November 2005). www.ers.usda.gov/AmberWaves/November05/DataFeature.

20. The chicken breast meal has about 731 calories; the gum drops, 721.

   One calorie measures the amount of energy required to raise the temperature of one gram of water (.035 ounce, less than ¼ teaspoon) 1°C (that is, 1.8°F). In the old days, chemists would put a piece of food in a sealed chamber, surround the chamber by water, burn the food to ashes, and measure how much the surrounding water increased in temperature. These days, we're talking about how much energy something can become once your body metabolizes it: as stamina, as bone-building, as endocrine secretions, as glucose to feed the brain, as fat stores in the body, as digestive elimination.

   Problem is, in contemporary food writing when we discuss calories, we're actually talking about kilocalories (that is, 1,000 calories). If we say 1% milk has 102 calories per cup, we actually mean it has 102 kilocalories per cup—or 102,000 calories. But over the years, we've lopped off those last zeros to label the whole thing *calories*.

21. M. Veldhorst, et al, "Protein-Induced Satiety: Effects and Mechanisms of Different Proteins," *Physiology and Behavior*, vol. 94, no. 2 (2008), pp. 300–307; and D. Paddon-Jones, et al., "Protein, Weight Management, and Satiety," *American Journal of Clinical Nutrition*, vol. 87, no. 5 (2008), pp. 1558S–1561S.

22. Dietary fiber (aka roughage) comes from plants. It absorbs excess water from the digestive system and allows food to continue on its journey through our bodies without getting bogged down. There are two types of fiber: soluble (dissolves in water) and insoluble (does not dissolve in water). *Both* are indigestible by humans. Soluble fiber does alter as it makes its way through the body, getting fermented by bacteria and becoming a gel that aids in motility (the rate at which food moves through the system). It also slows the absorption of glucose, may lower total blood cholesterol, and balances acidity in the digestive track. Sources include all beans, oats, barley, some fruits (plums, apples, pears, berries, and bananas), broccoli, carrots, potatoes, sweet potatoes, and onions. By contrast, insoluble fiber speeds foods through the system and adds necessary bulk, which alleviates constipation. Sources include corn, wheat, nuts, seeds, green beans, cauliflower, zucchini, celery, and the skins of potatoes, apples, pears, and tomatoes.

   Dietary proteins are either clumps of or isolated bits of amino acids, one of the essential building blocks of all living, organic matter, beans to beef. We cannot build muscle or maintain body health without protein. Although our bodies are able to synthesize some amino acids, there are nine so-called essential amino acids that we cannot make on our own without ingesting them in our food. Important sources include meats, nuts, grains, beans, seeds, fish, eggs, and most dairy products.

23. Also called saccharides, carbohydrates (a.k.a. carbs) are the body's most ready source of energy, found plentifully in all sorts of sugars (like honey, maple syrup,

and brown sugar), grains (wheat, rice), fruit, berries, and starchy vegetables (such as potatoes). There are naturally occurring carbs (in spinach, grapes, or wheat, for example) and refined carbs (white sugar, all-purpose flour, wine, molasses, etc.). But they all come from plants: sugar from cane or beets, honey from pollen, etc.

24. The brown rice and butter have about 534 calories; the candy bar, about 541.

25. J. E. Blundell, et al., "The Fat Paradox: Fat-Induced Satiety Signals Versus High Fat Overconsumption," *International Journal of Obesity and Related Metabolic Disorders*, vol. 19, no. 11 (1995), pp. 832–835.

26. Mihalyi Csikszentmihalyi, *Flow: The Psychology of Optimal Experience* (New York: Harper Perennial, 1990), p. 75.

Step 4: Detox Your Palate from Useless Salt, Fat, and Sugars

1. None more compelling than David A. Kessler, *The End of Overeating: Taking Control of the Insatiable American Appetite* (New York: Rodale, 2009).

2. There are two basic electrolytes in our bodies that control so much of what happens: sodium and potassium. We need more potassium than sodium, but these days we consume more sodium than potassium. See Nina Planck's *Real Food: What to Eat and Why* (New York: Bloomsbury, 2006), p. 234–238; or Marion Nestle's *What to Eat: An Aisle-by-Aisle Guide to Savvy Food Choices and Good Eating* (New York: North Point Press, 2006), pp. 365–367.

3. Karen McMahon, "What Is the Role of Salt in Taste?" *Proceedings of the 20th Workshop/Conference of the Association for Biology Laboratory Education*, vol. 20 (1999), pages 387–389.

4. "Americans Eat Too Much Salt, CDC Says," *Reuters*, May 26, 2009, www .reuters.com/article/healthNews/idUSTRE52P65820090326. Also see the USDA publication "Dietary Guidance on Sodium: Should We Take It with a Grain of Salt?" (May 1997) found at www.cnpp.usda.gov/publications/nutritioninsights/ insight3.pdf.

5. The forthcoming statistics are from "Sodium: Are You Getting Too Much?" in *Nutrition and Healthy Eating* at www.mayoclinic.com/health/sodium/NU00284.

6. Marion Nestle, *What to Eat* (New York: North Point Press, 2006), p. 125.

7. "U.S. Sweetener Consumption Trends and Dietary Guidelines," Iowa State University Center for Agricultural and Rural Development, Winter 2005, vol. 11, no. 1. www.card.iastate.edu/iowa_ag_review/winter_05/article5.aspx.

8. To be clear, Americans aren't eating 43 teaspoons of table sugar a day. Rather, this is the amount of all sweeteners converted into table sugar. Still, given that all sweeteners have about the same number of calories by weight, the modified numbers are valid.

9. See the USDA's "Briefing Room" on sugar and sweeteners at www.ers.usda.gov/Briefing/Sugar.

10. From the USDA's factbook, chapter 2, "Profiling Food Consumption in America," p. 20. See www.usda.gov/factbook/chapter2.pdf. There's a problem with the quote: it's not really *sugar* per se—unless we use a very broad definition of the word. Not all sweeteners are table sugar (as in the refined stuff, a.k.a. sucrose).

11. See Stephen H. Fairclough and Kim Houston, "A Metabolic Measure of Mental Effort," *Journal of Biological Psychology*, vol. 66, no. 2 (2004), pp. 177–190.

12. Studies cited in Gillian Harris, "Development of Taste Perception and Appetite Regulation" in *Infant Development: Recent Advances*, ed. Gavin Bremner, et al. (New York: Psychology Press, 1997), p. 18.

13. Phone conversation with Barbara J. Rolls, July 30, 2009.

14. Actually, they've been able to get it up to 90%, but the product is in limited supply and ghastly unpalatable.

15. By dry weight. See Table 29, "U.S. high fructose corn syrup (HFCS) production, quarterly, and by fiscal, and calendar year" in "Sugar and Sweeteners Yearbook Tables: Excel Spreadsheets" under "Sugar and Sweeteners: Recommended Data" on the USDA's website at www.ers.usda.gov/briefing/sugar/data.htm.

16. Some might object to our placing it here. "Why not in *not real food*? they might ask." Our journey is about pleasure and taste. In the complicated milieu of these sweeteners, refined sugar is a step in the right direction. There's no attempt to fake us out.

17. Marion Nestle, *What to Eat* (New York: North Point Press, 2006), p. 327.

18. This is a matter of weight, not volume. A teaspoon of sugar has about 15 calories; a teaspoon of heavier honey has more, depending on the variety.

Step 5: Take the Long View

1. Research from David Benton at Swansea University in the United Kingdom documents that infants have more open palates, fewer dislikes, when their environments are positive. When parents are themselves afraid of new things or hesitate before offering that bit of creamed spinach on a spoon, a baby is more likely to react negatively in kind—and (here's the kicker) to develop poor eating habits. Babies read nonverbal cues. They sense that fear—and mimic those cues. Fear breeds fear. The range of dislikes can soon overwhelm the few likes—and yes, the child then has a greater chance for obesity or eating disorders later in life. See D. Benton, "Role of Parents in the Determination of the Food Preferences of Children and the Development of Obesity," *International Journal of Obesity*, vol. 28, no. 7 (2004), pp. 858–869.

2. Indeed, compulsive overeating is often tied to boredom. See Laura Canetti, et al., "Food and Emotion" in *Behavioural Processes*, vol. 60, no. 2 (2002), p. 157–164; and for a more sustained treatment (if actually directed at adolescents), Judith Peacock, *Compulsive Overeating: Perspectives on Mental Health* (New York: LifeMatters, 2004). Boredom comes in many varieties—and being bored with what we're eating can also lead to overeating as we miss cues to satiety. For example, the same-old-sameness of much bland diet fare can lead to excessive eating. See Christine E. Howard and Linda Krug Porzelius, "The Role of Dieting in Binge Eating Disorder: Etiology and Treatment Implications," in *Clinical Psychology Review*, vol. 19, no. 1 (1999), pp. 24–44.

3. E-mails with Marion Nestle, July 29-August 1, 2009.

4. Any discussion of the seafood counter brings up the ongoing and difficult question of sustainability in fish stocks. If you'd like to keep tabs on the ongoing problem, download comprehensive sustainability lists to your computer or hand-held device from the Monterey Bay Aquarium (www.montereybayaquarium.org) or the Environmental Defense Fund (www.edf.org).

5. Perhaps the best single study followed a group of college students, asking them to become self-conscious about their eating habits (as well as other habits). These students in a mere matter of weeks showed increased self-control and better eating habits than the group left to their own devices. See Mark Muraven, et al., "Longitudinal Improvement of Self-Regulation Through Practice: Building Self-Control Strength Through Repeated Exercise," *Journal of Social Psychology*, vol. 139 (1999), pp. 446–457.

6. Condensed e-mail correspondence over several days with Joyce Hendley March 10 to March 16, 2009.

7. R. R. Wing and J. O. Hill, "Successful Weight Loss Management," in *Annual Review of Nutrition*, vol. 21 (2001), pp. 323–341.

Step 6: Upgrade Your Choices

1. A long-term study found that Americans get a minimal amount of whole grains each day; only eight percent of the population gets the recommended three servings of whole grains a day. See Linda E. Cleveland, et al., "Dietary Intake of Whole Grains," *Journal of the American College of Nutrition*, vol. 19, no. 90003 (2000), pp. 331S–388S.

2. A. Nilsson, et al., "Effects of GI and Content of Indigestible Carbohydrates of Cereal-Based Evening Meals on Glucose Tolerance at a Subsequent Standardized Breakfast," in *European Journal of Clinical Nutrition*, vol. 60, No. 60 (2006), pp. 1092–1099.

Step 7: Treat Yourself Well

1. Alex A. Kartashov, et al., "Eating Breakfast May Reduce Risk of Obesity, Diabetes, Hearth Disease," *The Science Blog*, March 8, 2003, at www.scienceblog.com/cms/eating_breakfast_may_reduce_risk_of_obesity_diabetes_heart_disease

2. Sungsoo Cho, et al., "The Effect of Breakfast Type on Total Daily Energy Intake and Body Mass Index: Results from the Third National Health and Nutrition Examination Survey (NHANES III)," *Journal of the American College of Nutrition*, vol. 22, no. 4 (2003), pp. 296–302.

3. Arlet V. Nedeltcheva, et al., "Sleep Curtailment Is Accompanied by Increased Intake of Calories from Snacks," *American Journal of Clinical Nutrition*, vol. 89, no. 1 (2009), pp. 126–133.

4. University of Chicago Medical Center, "New Study Shows People Sleep Even Less Than They Think," *ScienceDaily* (July 3, 2006), www.sciencedaily.com-/releases/2006/07/060703162945.htm.

Index

Gelling agents, 38–40
Ginger, 103
Glucose, 152–53, 156, 248
Goat Cheese and Peach Quesadillas, 14
Grains, 85, 199, 210–23, 248
  whole, 26, 61, 76, 105, 199, 210–23,
    224, 248, 249–51
  See also specific grains
Granola, 249, 255–56
Grass-fed, 233
Grilled Caesar Salad, 175
Grilled Fennel with Avocado Oil, 139
Guar gum, 39

Haddock with Vegetable Noodles,
    Broiled, 238–39
Ham, 61
Heart disease, 248
Herbs and spices, 11, 45–47, 200
  Herb-Stuffed Trout, 8
  Three Popcorn Spices, 257
  uses of, 46–54
  See also specific herbs and spices
High-fructose corn syrup, 155–57
Honey, 11, 161–63
  Banana Bread, 163–64
  Honey-Mustard Vinaigrette, 68
  types of, 161–62
Hormone-free, 233
Hot sauces, 76, 169
Hummus, Red Pepper, 137–38

Ice cream, 55
Imagination, 44

Jams and preserves, 76, 205
Journal, food, 201–208

Kosher salt, 128–29

Labels, food, 44–45, 62–63, 159
Laboratory, food, 35–41
Lamb:
  Braised Shanks with Lemon and
    White Beans, 112–13
  shopping for, 187–89

Lard, 144
Lecithin, 39
Leeks, 179
Lemon, 11
  Braised Lamb Shanks with White
    Beans and, 112–13
  Chicken Cutlets, 95–96
Lentil:
  Pear, and Walnut Salad, 106
  Red Lentil Stew, 127–28
Lettuce, 23, 24, 25, 178
Lobster, 98
Locust bean gum, 39
Lunch, 205–206, 252

Macaroni and Broccoli and Mushrooms
    and Cheese, Skillet, 106–108
Maple syrup, 164–65
  Walnut-Date Scones, 165–66
Mapo Dofu, 193–94
Marinara, 67
Mayonnaise, 76, 174
Meat(s), 15, 117, 224, 226
  burgers, 22–25, 121, 167–70
  deli, 186–87
  shopping for, 187–89
  See also specific meats
Meat Loaf, Turkey Vegetable, 228–29
Media, food, 174
Memories, food, 6–7
Methylcellulose, 39
Milk, 36, 55, 76, 189
Minestrone Burgers, 49–50
Modified starch, 40
Molasses, 157, 169
Monoglycerides, 40
Monosodium glutamate (MSG), 41, 123
More-Vegetable-Than-Meat Chili,
    227–28
Muesli, 251
Muffins, Refrigerator, 250
Multigrain Waffle Mix, 251
Mushroom(s), 168
  Chicken, Fennel, and Mushroom
    Casserole, 149–50
  Fettuccini with, 177